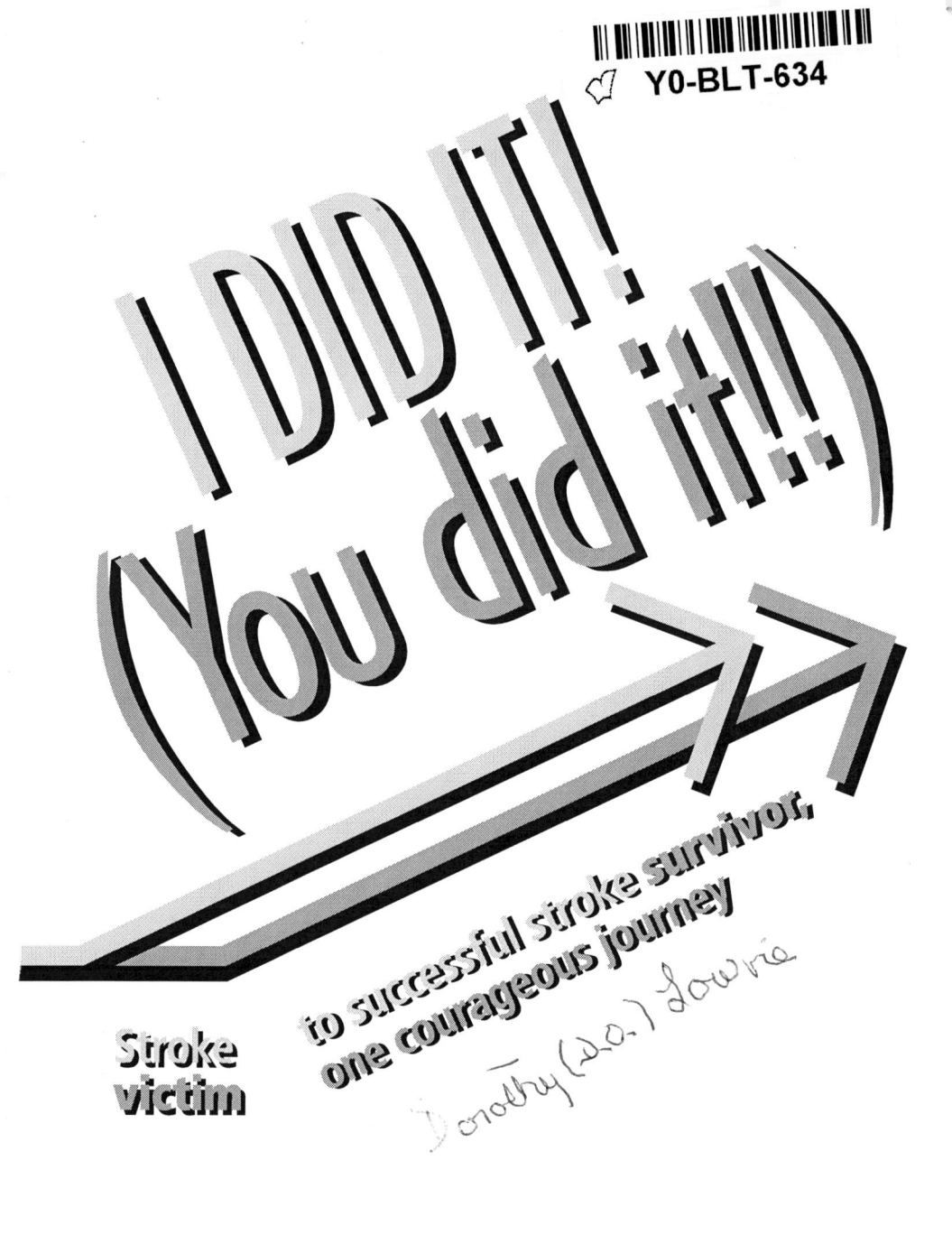

I DID IT!
(You did it!!!)

Stroke victim to successful stroke survivor, one courageous journey

Dorothy (D.O.) Lowrie

Stevia W. Sargent Lesher
Dorothy Williams Lowrie

I DID IT! (You did it!!)

"I DID IT! (You did it!!)" Copyright © 2004 Stevia W. Sargent Lesher and Dorothy Williams Lowrie. All rights reserved. Printed in the United States. No part of this book may be used or reproduced in any manner whatsoever without written permission except in critical articles and reviews. For information address Ms. S. Lesher, 5780 South Cherokee Street, Littleton, CO 80120-2339.

Cover design S.W.S.L.

Book graphic design: Image Illustration Studio, LLC. www.imageillustration.com.

Initial typing/editing: Patricia S. Perry.

Manuscript transcription: Accurate Business Services, Inc.

Publishers: Walter O. Lowrie and Stevia W. Sargent Lesher.

DEDICATION

To Walt, without whose steadfast love and encouragement I might not have persisted.

*   D.O.*

And to them both, D.O. and Walt: Bravo, well done!! Carry on.

*   Stevie*

I DID IT! (You did it!!)

ACKNOWLEDGEMENTS

Special mention and thanks go to those specialists who worked so hard with the people in this story:

Philip R. Yarnell, M.D., former Chairman: Department of Neurology, Denver General Hospital;

Mary Gosnell, R.P.T., Denver Physical Therapy Associates;

Patricia Monroe, R.S.T., former Chairman: Department of Speech Pathology, Denver General Hospital;

and to their counterparts everywhere who evidence such care and expend countless hours as they goad and guide in their particular fields.

We would also like to thank our families – particularly the younger Leshers – who endured periodic neglect during this writing project, and all those who aided and abetted the development of this manuscript: without their insights and encouragement this book would still be but a dream...

Pat Zollinger, Nancy Simon, Robert B. Perry, M.D., Patricia S. Perry, Kay Polsby, RN, Nancy Miani, Walter O. Lowrie, Barbara Kimball, Veronica Holt, Pamela Erickson, RN, Ann Berman, Lea W. Arabia, Marion Anson...Salud!

CONTENTS

PREFACE – Philip R. Yarnell, M.D.

INTRODUCTION

PROLOGUE

I	HOME AGAIN	1
II	BY THE END OF ONE WEEK	9
III	FRUSTRATIONS: Chores, Christmas, Places, Assumptions	31
IV	GAMES AND NON-GAMES	45
V	RESPONSIBILITY SHIFTS	69
VI	FORGING AHEAD	81
VII	SETBACKS	91
VIII	NEW TOYS, OLD PROBLEMS, AND INDEPENDENCE	99
IX	NOTES FROM JOURNAL, FEBRUARY 1977	111
X	EIGHT MONTHS LATER	113
XI	EPILOGUE	119
	ADDENDUM	131
	BOOK ORDERS	132
	AUTHORS	133

PREFACE

 This is a powerful, emotionally moving, true story told in two voices of the struggle to regain function and independence, after a devastating stroke. D.O., a 47-year-old vibrant, educated, active mother, homemaker, volunteer, and wife of a prominent corporate executive, was struck down with a dense right hemiplegia and severe mixed aphasia, at age 47. The cause, a left-middle cerebral artery occlusion, occurred without known risk factors. Stevie, a contemporary and an acquaintance of D.O. with her own family obligations, but needing a job, is hired to be D.O.'s rehabilitation aide/coordinator.

 In the process of her job, Stevie becomes a lay physical, occupational and speech therapist as well as a coach. She brings D.O. to her outpatient therapies. She then continues to work with the patient on her home program, as given by the therapists, plus improvisational additions, devised by her and D.O. The numerous vignettes: 1) trying to overcome spasticity with repetitive use, stretching, massage, biofeedback; 2) working to break through the Broca's type aphasia with mainly exercises and phrase completion and spontaneous speech with constant corrections, repetitions; 3) learning activities of daily living, including dressing, unscrewing bottle caps, and doing the laundry are documented in a most informative and touching manner. Stevie describes the events and details and D.O. then comments in a separate sense of what her thoughts were and how she felt while she had very marked limitations in expressive ability. These vignettes range from humorous to painful, tear-evoking episodes, but are always informative in terms of trying to move the patient forward in functional ability.

These two women become friends and co-combatants in D.O.'s fight to regain independence. Stevie relates the arduous task of prodding and badgering while D.O. notes the great difficulty in overcoming the fatigue and pain with the spasticity, and the embarrassment of being unable to speak her needs. Thus, we see the rehabilitation course from the therapists' and the family's viewpoints, as represented by Stevie and the patient's point of view of the same therapies in D.O.'s voice. D.O. recounts her anger, "Why did this happen to me?" Her frustration, "Why am I still not well at the six-month mark?" The gains of walking with an aide, then with the ankle-foot orthotic brace, then being able to eventually take off the brace; to obtaining driving lessons by gaining control of her right leg and foot, and finally regaining her driver's license are all noted. However, the setbacks with illness, depression, fatigue and then a postinfarction seizure with medication and side effects are also described.

As an acute care neurologist who then follows his patients through their long-term rehabilitation course, this story rings most true. It should serve as an inspiration to families and patients of what a supervised rehabilitation program can accomplish. I recommend it also to physicians and therapists to better comprehend the patient's efforts involved in trying to work with therapies. Be prepared to cry and to laugh as you learn about the efforts of these two special women.

Philip R. Yarnell, M.D.
Neurology and Rehabilitation
Denver, Colorado
October 2004

INTRODUCTION

This book is about the victim of a stroke and her rehabilitation. We hope it will be helpful to others – lay persons, professionals, stroke patients and their families – who are faced with a similar challenge in their own lives.

After the basic chapters were developed, they were read by the patient, Dorothy ("D.O.") Lowrie and her family. From there she and I had many sessions: she would read, verbally correct my spelling or syntax (originally she had not been able to speak more than a few words after her stroke, much less read or write), and then add her comments from the perspective of three years later. D.O.'s words appear in capital letters, indented.

We have omitted most specifics of physical exercises; any mentioned are included only to illustrate the types involved. They should not be imitated as they are potentially dangerous and should only be undertaken on the orders of a physician and under the supervision of a registered physical therapist; we believe that to do otherwise is foolhardy.

A word of caution: although D.O.'s stroke was considered "massive," this does not mean that others having "massive strokes" will progress in the same direction or to the same degree. There are many variables in rehabilitation (not the least of which is individual response to trauma/stress). Degrees of progress are not predictable even given similar brain damage. The most that can be said is "Don't Give Up Trying!"

To what extent do socio-economic factors contribute to (or detract from) a stroke rehabilitation program? We believe that financial ease (as in this case) is an "extra" and <u>not</u> a necessity for progress. What is important is a persistent attitude on the part of the patient <u>and</u> those immediately involved on a day-to-day basis. This was – and still is – the dominant factor with this stroke victim and her family.

Lest anyone think that planned activities always succeeded, they did not. There were occasions when D.O. was asked to try something which, at the time, was really impossible for her to accomplish. That particular activity was immediately dropped – and returned to in a different form weeks or months later, sometimes with success, sometimes not. Trial and error…but <u>always</u> Trial!

Stevia W. Sargent Lesher   Dorothy Williams Lowrie

I DID IT! (You did it!!)

PROLOGUE

"CVA" they call it – cerebrovascular accident, the third largest killer in the United States, with thousand of survivors each year. Stroke, that accident of trauma with paralysis, spasticity (or sometimes the extreme opposite, flaccidity), and communication problems to greater or lesser extents. Stroke – no warning, it just happened.

> THE MINUTE I WALKED INTO THE BOOKSTORE I REALIZED THAT SOMETHING WAS NOT RIGHT. I STUMBLED AND TRIED TO GET OUT OF THE WAY OF THE OTHER CUSTOMERS, AND CRUMPLED ON A PILE OF BOOKS. THE OWNER ASKED IF I WAS ALL RIGHT. AND I MUST HAVE PASSED OUT RIGHT THEN. THE NEXT THING I REMEMBER WAS A PART OF THE RIDE IN THE AMBULANCE, JUST A FLEETING MOMENT, AND THEN NOTHING UNTIL I WAS IN THE INTENSIVE CARE UNIT. MY HUSBAND SAYS THIS WAS AT LEAST TWO HOURS LATER, AFTER I HAD BEEN IN THE EMERGENCY ROOM. NO WAY CAN I REMEMBER THIS NOW, THOUGH.

"D.O." her friends call her, a nickname from childhood when young contemporaries could not say "Dorothy." I had known her socially for several years, and had by chance been hired by her to work for her mother who lived in a nursing home after several small strokes. Through the older lady's eyes I had glimpsed more of D.O. and her family. Occasionally, I was under the firm tutelage of a dynamic physical therapist who taught me how best to assist D.O.'s mother as she used her walker. The therapist and I had many conversations on disabilities, the do's and don'ts of helping people help themselves. No one could have imagined the value of those lessons.

News of D.O.'s stroke (at age forty-seven) traveled fast. It was a very real shock to everyone who knew her.

Five weeks later her husband called to see if I would be available to help out two to three hours a day when D.O. returned home from the rehabilitation center. Needing a job and glad to help someone who had helped me, I accepted. I had no specific qualifications, no medical or rehabilitation training. My only experience with a medical catastrophe had been with a male cousin, paraplegic after an auto accident two years earlier. Nor had I any inkling of the coming involvement in another's efforts to survive and to succeed. But I believed I certainly could help with household tasks, and that she and I would get along.

She was unusual, this woman I knew. Adjectives and phrases repeated as family and friends described her: intelligent, lovely, active; always doing for others: loving support and gracious hostess for successful executive husband; caring daughter of an ailing mother; warm mother to three grown children; leadership level volunteer and state-wide lobbyist; homemaker and partner. And now?

I called the physical therapist and found that she had already seen D.O. She told me the effects of the stroke. I did not comprehend the description she gave – nothing really prepared me for that reality. The therapist then set the stage for all the days to follow: "We must get her going." I had no idea what she meant, but these words stuck and were my first support as I later struggled to zero in on what had to be done.

Chapter I

HOME AGAIN

When I first saw D.O. six weeks after her stroke, I was appalled and completely unprepared. She could walk with a brace, but with great difficulty; slowly swinging her right leg around from her hip. Her right arm was almost always bent tight across her chest, and her right hand, badly swollen, was in a perpetual fist. No brightness was in her eyes. She was pale. She could hardly speak.

I could not bear to look at her right hand.

She experienced nearly constant pain in her right hand and shoulder with unpredictable spasms: breath-catching, tear-producing pain. We were helpless, there was nothing to do but let her try different positions by using her left hand to move her right arm.

A left-sided stroke in the brain meant, for D.O., partial paralysis of her right limbs ("right hemiplegia.") Patches of her face were numb, and her taste was altered. Some foods she had enjoyed before her stroke were now inedible.

She had severe expressive aphasia and some apraxia, terms I later learned indicate literal memory loss of words and some loss of mouth-tongue muscle control in the formation of words (or even in whistling). Her right foot, without the brace, was spastic: it turned down and in. It, too, was painful.

But she was up and dressed. Six weeks earlier no one knew whether she would even live. She had learned the art of eating and dressing with her left hand. It was still hard however, for her to put on her stockings, and the brace was a real challenge because of the spasticity of her right foot and her tight heel cord. The shoe was attached to the brace, and positioning her foot into it was a task. Once in, and the strap holding the side metal struts fastened just below her knee, the brace maintained her foot at a right angle to her leg so that she could walk.

> WHEN I FIRST CAME HOME, I DON'T KNOW HOW MY HUSBAND STOOD IT: EVERY NIGHT I WOULD START TO SAY SOMETHING, AND I COULDN'T SAY IT, AND I WOULD CRY AND CRY.

She sat. The one thing she did voluntarily those first days at home was to get up slowly, walk eight feet, and let the dogs out or in.

Her reasoning abilities were still intact, but other communication functions were badly affected. She could hear normally, but could not always comprehend what people were really saying; and the processing of words and thoughts – something we all do automatically – was often confused and inaccurate. She no longer understood the meaning of abstract information and her retention was moderately impaired. But by far her biggest problem was linguistic: naming, word choice,

Chapter I — Home Again

usage and grammatical abilities were almost non-existent. With effort D.O. said "yes" and "no" and one word comments or desires. Even "yes" and "no" were sometimes transposed.

> YOU WILL NEVER KNOW HOW AWFUL IT IS NOT TO BE ABLE TO TALK. IN THOSE FIRST FEW WEEKS, IT WAS ALL I COULD DO TO SAY ANYTHING. I DID NOT REALIZE THAT I WAS SWITCHING "YES" FOR "NO" (OR VICE VERSA), AND WHEN YOU OR ANYONE ACTED ON MY FALSE ANSWERS, I THOUGHT YOU WERE NUTS. WHEN YOU EXPLAINED WHAT I HAD SAID, I WAS APPALLED AND HUMILIATED. YOU WOULD APOLOGIZE, AND THEN ASK ME THE SAME QUESTION ALL OVER AGAIN. ONLY, THIS TIME, YOU WOULD DOUBLE CHECK MY ANSWER AND I SEETHED INSIDE; BUT I WAS SECRETLY AFRAID THAT WHAT I HAD SAID WAS INCORRECT AGAIN.

We were nervous, she and I. Seeing a vital 47-year-old reduced to this physical and verbal condition was shattering – and guilt-producing. The "why-did-this-happen-to-her" made no sense, despite my basic belief that there <u>is</u> always a reason (even if I don't always know what it is). It was all I could do to try to mask my horror and sadness. Surely she would not be this way forever? What could I <u>do</u>? What could I <u>say</u>? <u>What</u>?

> I WAS HAPPY TO BE HOME, JUST TO BE HOME. I WAS HAPPY TO THINK ABOUT THANKSGIVING COMING SOON. BUT, OF COURSE, THERE WAS A

GENERAL FRUSTRATION LEVEL WHENEVER I THOUGHT "I WANT TO DO" WHATEVER IT WAS AND COULD NOT PHYSICALLY DO IT OR NECESSARILY SAY IT FOR THAT MATTER. AND I WAS REALLY ANGRY THAT I COULD HEAR THE TENNIS PLAYERS JUST DOWN THE ROAD: I USED TO BE ON THE COURT ALMOST EVERY DAY, TOO, AND NOW EVERYBODY ELSE BUT ME WAS PLAYING. I WAS ANGRY.

We tried to talk. Anything, everything. Basic questions about her past which, although we had been casual friends for several years, I had never bothered to ask. I asked now so that she could answer with a nod, "yes" or "no" school, college, major, marriage, work, children, dogs, weather, coffee? ("Yes".) And, inappropriately, she laughed – or cried – with no clue as to why, it just came and sometimes melded one into the other. A normal laugh (or cry) was grossly exaggerated, almost hysterical. No one knew whether she was really happy (or sad) and she could not speak well enough to tell us. Josh, coddle, laugh became my routine to stop these outbursts. Politics, neighbors, dogs, children…Talk!

On this first day her eldest daughter was home from work. She smoothed the familiarization process of a near stranger, showing me those essentials of D.O.'s home. More than that, she set the tone, interpreting her mother's speech attempts, comforting the outbursts of tears without undue concern or emotion. And when her mother went for an extended nap after

Chapter I — Home Again

lunch, it was to this daughter that I turned to ask questions about D.O.'s pre-stroke activities and interests.

I knew that these questions might be painful for the daughter, but I was already resolving to do whatever I could to help. With D.O.'s communication skills so badly impaired, I tried to find out as much as possible as quickly as possible so that later I could ask her these same questions with a reasonable certainty of correctly interpreting her answers. Believing that life is a continuum, I wanted to know more about the past so that threads could be woven into the present and future.

> YOU DIDN'T KNOW – AND I COULDN'T TELL YOU – WHAT MY SPEECH PROBLEMS WERE, AND WHO BUT THOSE WHO HAD HAD EXPERIENCE WITH APHASIA COULD BELIEVE THAT WORDS HAD QUITE LITERALLY DISAPPEARED FROM MY MIND? OR, IF THEY WERE THERE, THAT I COULD NOT SAY THEM?
>
> I KNEW A CHAIR WAS A CHAIR; BUT WHEN YOU WENT AROUND THE ROOM ASKING ME TO NAME OBJECTS, I COULD NOT DO IT. IT WAS DEVASTATING, FRIGHTENING, AND MADDENING ALL AT THE SAME TIME. BUT I KNEW THAT I WAS BETTER THAN I HAD BEEN IN THE HOSPITAL.

The following day I asked D.O. if she could read. "No." I wondered: does she mean "yes?" Surely she could read, this super-bright gal who normally did the New York Times crossword puzzle in jig time. I searched for a child's book and showed it to her. Nothing. She just shook her head. She could not read. Empty pit in my stomach; cover up fast. "Coffee?" I asked. "Yes."

I became intrigued with these problems and the challenge of building on those few words which she could say. A few days later D.O. showed me a notebook she had had in the rehabilitation center. It had pages of word exercises, short sentences in large print which lacked one or two words. She had been able to fill in the missing words properly, usually using the most complex word for an object ("automobile" for "car," for example). Obviously she could, indeed, read. But that skill was extremely limited and depended on size, length of the material, and help. She could not read a normal page of print; she told me months later that the words all ran together, no matter how hard she tried to separate them.

Based on the written exercises, I started to "cue" her: instead of asking D.O. to name the chair, for instance, I asked her to finish my phrase "you are sitting on the _____"; or "I would like a cup of _____." She could speak these words, (chair, coffee) when cued this way.

I began to encourage her to do something "new" each day, something she had not tried since coming home. The exact activity mattered little as long as she made the effort. We walked to the mailbox, about forty feet down the driveway. Step, swing-drag, step. It took half an hour. Mutual pleasure that she walked so far. She was exhausted.

Chapter I   —   Home Again

Naps and rests were mandatory. She usually slept two hours in the afternoons, with frequent five to ten minute quiet periods during the day. I had to learn that in doing anything she now expended enormous brain energy. She had to think over and work out each movement ahead of time to take into account the paralysis/spasticity of her right arm and partial paralysis of her right leg. Even before arising in the morning, she had to organize her thoughts based on these new realities. No more could she just get up and walk. And as I learned later, most handicapped persons dream of themselves as they were before their illness or injury. Waking up, therefore, forced daily and immediate realization of handicaps: mentally, emotionally and physically. I watched for tiredness. It was real yet not always realized by her.

The spasms and pain continued with no forewarning. Specialists in speech and physical therapy beckoned – specialists selected by D.O. and her husband before her return home. Her husband asked if I could drive her to and from these appointments. Quickly agreeing, my hours of work lengthened as D.O. committed herself to the continuation of those formalized re-learning sessions. Rehabilitation.

Chapter II

BY THE END OF ONE WEEK

I was now working nearly full time. Tentative schedules were arranged with the therapists: five sessions a week with the physical therapist, and three times a week with the speech therapist. These trips in themselves were tiring and took half an hour of driving each way.

On the third such trip there was a lengthy conference. The neurologist, the specialists, D.O. and I were all together for the first time to share opinions and courses of therapy for the coming months. It was at this point that my working an eight-hour day was suggested in order for there to be maximum follow-through at home.

The specialists bantered terminology and techniques, and I took notes of unknown words and strategies to be referenced later for clarity. They all were in basic agreement: D.O. must work as much as possible each day, five days a week. Activity was vital: she must be kept busy doing and thinking. A schedule must develop whereby specifics would be required – a structured environment to allow opportunity for the greatest mental and physical stimulation and the greatest progress. Evenings should be relaxation with her family. Weekends would not be totally "free." Some speech and physical exercises would have to be done on her own.

The ride home was quiet that day as I began to adjust to my developing role in this rehabilitation effort. It was scary, it was challenging. And, for whatever reason, we did not discuss the coming days except in relation to the tasks which would be asked of her.

The silence was unusually long; I sensed another "low."

Every day D.O. had one or more short periods of depression. Sometimes she cried, sometimes not, but it was obvious whenever she felt overwhelmed. The profound shock, frustration and fear following a stroke compounded the struggles of any activity, and swings in mood were many and to be expected. I tried to be aware of each occurrence of depression, and to let her know that I realized the psychological pain she was experiencing. I comforted as best I could with an arm around her shoulders or a pat on her head, and mumbled those words of "I know, you're all right, it will be all right," quickly shifting the emphasis to how much she was loved and counted on by her family, how much we all expected of her, and how well she was doing. I tried to limit these periods to not more than a few minutes, and always signaled their end with an amusing anecdote and with something specific we had to do right then.

> I DON'T KNOW WHY MY HUSBAND DIDN'T DIVORCE ME. FOR SEVERAL MONTHS I FELT SO USELESS, AND I CRIED OFTEN. I EVEN THOUGHT OF SUICIDE. I JUST DIDN'T KNOW HOW I WAS GOING TO PULL THROUGH.

Chapter II — By the end of one week

I HAD RECURRENT DOUBTS ABOUT WHETHER I WOULD EVER BE USEFUL AGAIN, WHETHER I WOULD EVER BE ABLE TO COPE WITH ANYTHING AGAIN NOW THAT EVERYTHING HAD CHANGED SO DRASTICALLY. LOOKING BACK, I HAD THESE LOW PERIODS SEVERAL TIMES A DAY AT FIRST, BUT THEY CAME LESS OFTEN AFTER 3-4 MONTHS. TODAY MY "LOWS" ARE NOT AS EXTREME AND ARE MORE NORMAL IN TERMS OF FREQUENCY. BUT, IN THE BEGINNING, I WAS IN BAD SHAPE PSYCHOLOGICALLY.

EVERYONE WAS KIND AND EMPATHETIC WHENEVER I WAS DEPRESSED. BUT THEY KNEW THAT IT WAS NOT GOOD FOR ME TO DWELL ON MY PROBLEMS FOR LONG PERIODS OF TIME. HAVING SO MUCH TO DO EVERY DAY WAS A NATURAL BARRIER TO THE LENGTH OF THOSE DEPRESSIONS.

The days' schedules were quickly organized, and we made sure that on some days we could stop and have lunch out, a break between therapy sessions. Curbs, revolving doors, and elevator doors are unavoidable and I became "defensive guard" on a sidewalk or in a restaurant in case someone unwittingly bumped into her. Ordering lunch was a game of "Sixty-four Questions" in which my assumptions were not always accurate; but each new challenge met received the praise of smiles. Progress – and on to the next specialist.

While at the hospital for Speech Therapy we ran into personnel D.O. knew from her stay there right after her stroke. Once an Occupational Therapist visited her in the speech room. Neither of us was at all prepared for her aggressiveness: the O.T. said hello and without further words grabbed D.O.'s right hand. The pain was immediate. D.O. moaned aloud. I was rooted to the floor in horror. D.O. said "no – no – no" but was unable to explain why: my words were little more coherent as I stammered the obvious: her hand was still swollen, spastic and painful all the time and could <u>not</u> be grabbed. The O.T., still aggressive, finally released D.O.'s hand and left. D.O. was flabbergasted – and the incident was imprinted on my mind as one example of the insensitivity of some who, because of their professions, should have been trained to observe more closely and have a "feel" for a situation.

I was given specific instructions for when we were at home: speech exercises, physical exercises, and ways to try doing things differently. There was always more to be done than was feasible. Pressure.

Continuing motivation. Alternative pressure so that there were periods when nothing was demanded. Driving was my time to chat – to comment on things we passed, to enlarge the focus world-wide to issues and activities elsewhere. Watching T.V. was relaxation for D.O.; she watched it every night.

> IT WAS NO PROBLEM TO WATCH T.V. AND TO ABSORB, BUT I COULD NOT RE-TELL IT NO MATTER HOW HARD I TRIED.

Chapter II — By the end of one week

One word answers, sometimes.

Joke – about friends we have in common, about my children sneaking our goat into the living room to surprise unwary guests, joke about anything! And, after a week of grueling schedules and near monologues, the day came when <u>she</u> initiated speech as the stoplight turned green: "Go!" (Once, several weeks later, she repeated this gambit and was told that no longer was this acceptable speech, she could do better than that for-God's-sake. Hurt – and pride that progress was recognized – and no more simple "Go's" at stoplights!)

Before I entered her home every morning I stopped, mentally counted to 20, and took a deep breath. I reminded myself to slow down my speech and movement. And I lectured myself: I must wait for her to speak, to try to finish her own sentences and thoughts. The patience factor was critical for the recovery of her speech and orderly thoughts. We all knew this, although sometimes we, too, forgot.

> THE ONLY TIMES I GOT REALLY ANGRY WERE WHEN I WAS ABOUT TO SAY SOMETHING REALLY TREMENDOUS AND YOU CUT ME OFF. TODAY, IF PEOPLE CUT ME OFF – MY SPEECH IS STILL SLOW SOMETIMES – I SAY "WAIT A MINUTE, I'M NOT FINISHED." BUT, TODAY I CAN SAY THAT.

"Fifteen minutes" she said when she could not find or say an answer to a question (meaning "Give me fifteen minutes and I will be able to answer you," sometimes she did, sometimes she didn't). The frustrations of lack of speech are unbelievable – and there were constant mix-ups and misunderstandings among us all.

For certain periods during the day, D.O. now wore a brace for her right wrist.

> HAVING TO WEAR THAT WAS CRUEL: THE COCK-UP OF MY RIGHT HAND WAS UNBELIEVABLE, IT HURT SO MUCH. AND BECAUSE OF THE SPASTICITY IN MY WRIST AND HAND, I COULD BARELY GET THE BRACE ON. BUT SOMEHOW I MANAGED BECAUSE I HAD TO. WHEN I RECALL THE AGONY I WONDER: "WHY DID I BOTHER?"

Spasticity and pain were always at a high level with this procedure, as was her frustration. The brace forced her hand up higher than her wrist. The pain of the least upward pressure on her right hand was excruciating. Without the brace, however, there was a good possibility that tendons in her wrist would be permanently tight and her hand forever a claw.

One time she stood in the kitchen trying to get the brace on, and then could not understand (or say) why her daughter or I hadn't got her coat. We were late for a therapy appointment. Tears and anger. To the car. Once driving, I took her back to the situation and explained how we had been involved in her agony with the wrist brace; neither her daughter nor I had known that she wanted her coat. The humor of the situation hit her; she laughed.

She could and did laugh – with others and at herself. But all the time the over-riding thought: "I've got to get well, I've got to

Chapter II — By the end of one week

get better, and I've got to try."

My gradual transition from casual friend/helper to the enforcer of specific tasks and exercises was relatively smooth, and made easier because I, too, was accountable to the specialists. As in a one-man play, I acted a variety of roles to get the job done and did not hesitate to over-exaggerate my middle position whenever D.O. balked at my directions. "I'm going to get in trouble if you don't do what we are supposed to do." Sure enough, when orders were not followed, it was I who was chastised by the specialists, in front of D.O. This sharing of responsibility worked well: each of us was under the gun to perform.

I took voluminous notes on speech and physical exercises as they were demonstrated by the specialists, and practiced them in the office to make sure I understood the correct procedures. Additionally, I scribbled particulars from each session – where D.O. did well, or where there was need for more exercise or drilling. I wrote four to five pages a day, partly during these therapy sessions and the rest added late at night with more details of daily events, reactions and discussions. Each morning I read the previous day's pages, and made a list of "must do's" to remind myself of all the pieces which we had to fit into the next eight hours.

> EIGHT HOURS? BE SERIOUS: SOMETIMES YOU WERE HERE FOR TEN! YOU REFUSED TO LEAVE UNTIL EVERYTHING WAS DONE!

Physical exercises were real work, and sometimes quite painful. They were preceded, initially, by hot packs to loosen and relax tight tendons and muscles; later by cold packs to temporarily numb specific muscle groups which, when stretched or exercised, were very painful. The progress of getting down – and up again – from the floor was its own challenge: she could not do it unassisted, and I was terrified that I would not be able to hold her, that she would fall. We talked logistics before the first attempt, and by the next day she had a plan whereby she used the sofa and coffee table to support her; it worked.

Her every endeavor was praised, whether it was the first time she could raise her right leg off the floor half an inch, or learning to tie her shoelaces with her left hand; or saying "Good Morning, how are you?" all together. Everything had to be noticed and acknowledged. While she sometimes shrugged off compliments, inside they became further stimuli to try, to work, to improve. And once something was done, somehow, by herself, then it was never again done for her.

My natural inclination was to be on her right (affected) side whenever we were walking or trying something new. To my horror I found that just touching her right arm or armpit (much less her right hand) caused an immediate spasm of pain. And it was little use to grab an arm which did not respond. After several misguided attempts to be of help up curbs or down to the floor for exercises, I finally learned the habit of being next to her left (unaffected) side, feeling stupid at my initial clumsiness.

Chapter II   —   By the end of one week

Visitors and friends started to come over. It was a struggle to monitor who and how often, and to arrange, tactfully, for short visits. D.O. quietly bridled at my interception. It was a stressful time with her speech so limited. I was usually present to divert attention and provide a few minutes of non-speaking relief for her; and to reassure all that she <u>was</u> doing <u>well</u>, that her reasoning powers were still intact. And, as I walked these visitors to their cars, I absorbed some of their distress about D.O. having had a stroke and her present condition.

D.O. and I talked (I talked) about friends and reactions to seeing her. I tried to explain the guilt syndrome which I had to master – the "I'm glad it happened to you, not me" and immediate horror at such a thought. I suggested that it was up to her to let others know that she was "O.K." (By doing so she reinforced this belief within herself.) She was understanding and saw the point of putting others at ease; her responsibility was accepted and acted upon.

Visitors invariably told her how well she looked (she <u>was</u> looking better) and then jabbered away about their activities. And sometimes there was the "I know so-and-so with a stroke" comparison, or "Have you tried xyz?" Meaning to help, but helpless.

> WHEN FRIENDS CAME TO VISIT I WAS BOTH GRATEFUL AND EMBARRASSED. AS A MATTER OF FACT, ANY TIME ANYONE CAME UNEXPECTEDLY I WAS ON THE FLOOR WITH HOT OR COLD PACKS TOWELED TIGHT AROUND ME,

OR DOING EXERCISES. FRIENDS SAID, "IF THERE IS ANYTHING WE CAN DO, LET US KNOW." I WAS GRATEFUL, BUT THERE WAS LITTLE THEY COULD DO. I WAS REALLY VERY UNCOMFORTABLE WITH THEM, AND I THINK THEY WERE UNCOMFORTABLE WITH ME.

I HAD FEARS THAT I WAS MERELY TOLERATED BY EVERYBODY. I SUPPOSE I STILL HAVE TO WORK THIS THROUGH. TODAY, IF WE ARE GOING TO A LARGE PARTY AND THERE ARE MANY WHOM I KNOW CASUALLY, I AM TORN BETWEEN "THEY ARE NICE TO ME BECAUSE I AM HANDICAPPED" AND "THEY REALLY CARE." THIS IS STILL A HANG-UP, BUT I'M WORKING ON IT. I HAD NO PROBLEM, THOUGH, WITH GOING OUT IN PUBLIC.

It was a helpless feeling; people didn't know, couldn't know what to say, how or when to help. We all got caught, trying to help and only making things worse.

The tendency to supply a phrase or finish a sentence for her was natural. Yet she would not communicate better unless <u>she</u> figured it out, unless <u>she</u> talked. And it was frustrating to have someone else "helping" her speak, misjudge what it was she was trying to say; it was embarrassing for everyone as D.O. quickly shook her head "no" to another's finished sentence.

Every morning I asked her to tell me what she had done the previous evening, trying to prod her memory and to elicit sequential, structured speech.

Chapter II — *By the end of one week*

"I WAS TIRED."

When?

"YOU LEFT."

What? You're missing a word.

"BEFORE — NO, WHEN YOU LEFT."

Okay.

"I SAT. I ATE DINNER."

What did you have?

"OH – FISH – AND A GREEN VEGETABLE."

Please say that word again….a green <u>what</u>?

"VE / GE / TA / BLE."

Okay. Then?

"I RELAXED. I RETIRED."

What? Can you explain that?

"WENT TO BED!"

Who?

"I DO….DID."

What about your family?

"NATURALLY MY FAMILY IS HOME."

We are talking about last night – past tense, please.

"OH. MY FAMILY IS, NO…WAS PRESENT."

Okay. Was there anything unusual weather-wise?

"THE WHITE…NO. THE CLOUDS…WHAT DO YOU SAY?"

Do you mean "it snowed?"

"NO. THERE WAS A SNOWSTORM."

It was easier for her to start with the word "I." As when children first talk, the self was the most important and everything was visualized and remembered in this context. As D.O. did things during the day, she was supposed to verbalize whatever the action, to herself and out loud, starting with "I" (e.g. "I wake up," or "I get up," "I brush my teeth," "I get dressed" or "I am getting dressed," etc.) Several times each day I stopped whatever she was doing and asked her to describe it.

> I WAS OUTRAGED WHEN YOU TRIED TO MAKE ME TELL YOU WHAT I WAS DOING. I KNEW PERFECTLY WELL WHAT I WAS DOING – AS DID YOU – AND I FELT FOOLISH TALKING TO MYSELF. YOU KNOW WHAT? I DIDN'T DO IT ALOUD VERY OFTEN. I COULD HAVE SCREAMED WHEN YOU DEMANDED THESE DESCRIPTIONS: IT WAS ALL SO OBVIOUS, AND ELEMENTARY. BUT I COULD NOT ALWAYS SAY WHATEVER IT WAS, AND THAT MADE ME EVEN MADDER.

Chapter II — By the end of one week

She began to say some of those customary social niceties, each phrase pre-thought or rearranged in mid-saying whenever a particular word was missing from her vocabulary or came out sounding garbled. Sometimes she said words or phrases which made no sense. Usually, she heard the error and laughed, or, failing to realize what she had said, she was quick to catch my incredulous 'WHAT?" or my own giggles:

"THE DOG HAS BUTTERFLIES" (Meaning "The dog itches.")

"I WANT FRAGRANT MILK." (Meaning "I want a glass of milk."),

"SEE THE BEARS!" (Meaning "See the traffic!")

But D.O. could not correct these nonsensical verbalizations even if she knew the words she had used were wrong. For me, it became a fast mental game of hop, skip and jump to figure out what in the world she meant, and then to compose a phrase which might cue her well enough so that she could really say whatever it was by herself. It was not enough to be aware only of her: I had to know what was going on all around her – the birds, squirrels, street traffic, weather changes, strange dogs on the property, all household happenings; only in this way could I leap from the ridiculous "butterflies" to the intended "itches."

The speech therapist advised her to think through what she wanted to say, and then try to verbalize it. And whenever D.O. got stuck repeating an inaccurate beginning sound for a word, she was told to stop, easy does it, think of something else and come back to that particular word at a later time. A pause was less noticeable than a stammering: keep cool.

She began to learn word-substitution and reorganization of words. With an unusually large pre-stroke vocabulary and excellent visual sense, she worked through each question or response. It was work, nothing was automatic. And it was often trial and error. I used the dictionary frequently to check on the definitions of some exotic word she used, and found that she was usually correct in its usage. But, prepositions and verbs were her verbal Armageddon: often she said everything else, and then we went back and explored possible "in's" or "on's" or verbs she could have used. Synonyms took on an extra importance. We drilled and drilled, sometimes while she was lying still on the floor with cold packs on her right arm and hand.

The logs are (in) the fireplace.

The car is (in) the driveway.

My foot is (on) the floor.

The table is (next to) the chair.

Your brace is (on) your leg.

The newspaper is (in, on) your lap.

My blouse goes (over) my head.

Whenever possible I acted out these sentences with appropriate motions as visual cueing and reinforcement. The

Chapter II — By the end of one week

book, for example, was moved all around a table so that D.O. would say "over," "on," "beside," "under." These prepositions were misused often, and I laughed aloud when the book was "<u>in</u> the table." "No," I said, "it isn't <u>in</u> the table. Try it again."

When her patience was exhausted, D.O. would order: "Oh put the book -------." Forgetting the word "down" she took a breath and substituted "away."

The communication skill of re-telling something seen or heard became another mental exercise: this is what we all do in talking and was exceptionally hard for D.O. She was beginning to be able to read normal-sized print again, although reading aloud was very slow and some words were mispronounced. Occasionally she would substitute her own word for the printed word: New Orleans for New York, or shawl became sweater. She did not necessarily hear these substitutions, and they were usually akin to the actual word or subject area being discussed or read.

Each day D.O. now picked out a small article in the newspaper, cut it out, and put it in a special notebook, underlined the key words, looked up synonyms for these words, then read the article aloud. Then, book closed, I asked her to tell me about the article and what she thought about it. My, what progress in a few short weeks!

She did not like being corrected, and was trying to monitor herself and then self-correct. A tape recorder was put to use for reading aloud and some drills. It allowed her to hear her own mistakes, and was a good tool for sharpening her awareness of these errors. D.O. did not appreciate its use.

We battled over "to" or "toward," over grammar, over syntax. We battled over the number of verbs one could use when talking, for example, about a car – and she laughed at some of the resultant mental images.

> I REMEMBER THAT DRILL WELL. YOU WOULD SAY "I BLANK THE CAR," AND I HAD TO MAKE UP SENTENCES AND USE AS MANY VERBS AS I COULD…I SEE THE CAR. I DRIVE THE CAR. I WASH THE CAR. I STEER THE CAR. I PACK THE CAR. AND I UNPACK THE CAR. I PARK THE CAR. I SMASH THE CAR (smile). I DITCH THE CAR. I BORROW THE CAR. I SELL THE CAR. I BUY THE CAR. ETC. AND WHEN I COULD NOT THINK OF ANOTHER THING, YOU WOULD MAKE UP SITUATIONS WITH A CAR AND I WOULD HAVE TO COME UP WITH MORE VERBS. FOR EXAMPLE, YOU WOULD SAY "AND IN THE WINTER WHEN IT IS VERY COLD, YOU DO WHAT WITH THE CAR BEFORE DRIVING OFF?" FOR THAT ONE I REMEMBER SAYING "I HEAT THE CAR." YOU LAUGHED AND SAID, "I CAN SEE YOU TAKING A HEATER OUT TO QUOTE HEAT THE CAR." IT WAS FUNNY AND MADDENING AT THE SAME TIME IN THAT I COULD NOT ALWAYS SAY WHAT I REALLY WANTED TO SAY.
>
> THOSE DRILLS WERE AWFUL. AND I HATED TO SEE YOU GETTING THAT BLACK NOTEBOOK YOU

Chapter II   —   By the end of one week

KEPT FOR SPEECH EXERCISES: HERE WE GO AGAIN, I WOULD THINK, WHEN ALL I WANTED WAS A FEW MOMENTS OF PEACE.

Gradually she was standing up for herself, being surer of herself. She was developing new coping mechanisms. And when frustrations overwhelmed her, I became her whipping post: nothing I did or said was right. Her anger was subtle: seldom did she raise her voice or yell; instead, it was exhibited as an intellectual snub, a superiority against which I was helpless. Her intellect <u>was</u> far superior to the elementary speech and tasks we had to do, and I was secretly pleased that, despite her handicaps, she <u>knew</u> she was mentally far more capable. I absorbed, walked on eggs. The dogs were invaluable, providing amusement and love for her as well as relief for me as I threw balls for them outside, trying to recollect my wits and my humor.

A typical day's schedule left little time alone for herself:

EVERY DAY'S SCHEDULE WASN'T ANY PROBLEM, ALL OF IT JUST HAD TO BE DONE AND YOU AND I REALIZED IT. ON THE OTHER HAND, IF YOU HAD NOT BEEN HERE, I DON'T THINK I WOULD HAVE EVER GOTTEN OUT OF BED. I DON'T MEAN THAT I WOULD NOT HAVE FIXED DINNER OR LET THE DOGS IN AND OUT…PATRICIA NEAL SAID IN HER BOOK THAT SHE FELT LIKE A "PINK CABBAGE" AFTER HER STROKE; THAT IS A GOOD DESCRIPTION. I REALLY DO NOT KNOW WHAT I WOULD HAVE DONE ALL BY MYSELF, AND

NOBODY GAVE ME A CHANCE TO FIND OUT, EVEN THOUGH THERE WERE TIMES WHEN I WAS MADDER THAN HELL AT HAVING TO GET UP AND DO ALL THOSE THINGS.

I LOVE MY FAMILY – AND THEY WERE LOVELY AND CONCERNED, AND INTERESTED. BUT THEY ARE FAMILY. NO WAY COULD THEY TAKE THE PLACE OF AN OUTSIDER. BECAUSE YOU DID NOT HAVE THOSE FAMILIAL TIES AND MEMORIES, YOU COULD BE MORE OBJECTIVE, AND COULD SAY AND DO THINGS MY FAMILY COULD NOT. STEVIE, YOU KNOW WHAT WE WENT THROUGH, YOU AND I; <u>YOU</u> WERE UNUSUAL.

Unusual, too, was the family in their acceptance of the pressure we all had to put on her. They participated as much as the rest of us, and never once questioned my tactics or demands.

Determination: we all had it, her husband and children, her physician and therapists. Most of all, herself. As I told D.O. two years later: "Sure we were there with pitchforks, sure we pushed you beyond belief in those early stages and you had little choice but to do four hours' worth of exercises. But, as you progressed, as self-confidence redeveloped, NO ONE could have done anything without your tacit cooperation." D.O. knew this, but it was another needed compliment.

We became cohorts as students in a classroom, practicing sentences and exercises before seeing the therapists. We were "in cahoots" (a tactic which enables more practice – and progress!)

Chapter II — By the end of one week

I told the specialists of D.O.'s daily new accomplishments: of learning how to wash her hair with her left hand; of tying her coat-belt with one hand and her teeth; of one-handed use of the electric can opener. I told them that she had gone out for dinner with her husband and mastered a circular staircase up <u>and</u> down; that she sang old songs and had the words come automatically. (This is a normal phenomenon, I learned later, for those with aphasia: rote phrases are sometimes still automatic. This does not mean, however, that answers can be constructed or spoken clearly, or that basic comprehension functions normally.) She now went grocery shopping and was amazed at price changes in two months – and had trouble making decisions on items to buy.

Because I was with her every weekday, eight hours a day, and we faced the therapists together, D.O. had to answer honestly when they asked about her activities…

Yes, she was trying to ride the stationary bike daily;

No, she had not tried making cookies;

Yes, she was trying to watch the news on T.V. and talk about it;

Yes, she was using the tape recorder while doing some speech drills;

No, she had not done her explanation of proverbs that day.

"We have to do the proverb," I pleaded when we got home.

"Now's the time. Please tell me what this means: "Saying and Doing are Two Different Things."

> "SAYING YOU WILL DO IT — UH — IS SOMETHING THAT — UH — WE ALL DO AND — UH — LOTS OF PEOPLE SAY THEY'LL DO IT WITHOUT — UH — DOING IT BUT DOING SOMETHING IS ENTIRELY DIFFERENT — HEY, STEVIE, PLEASE READ THAT BACK TO ME."

I read it back, and then asked her to try explaining the proverb again.

> "LOTS OF PEOPLE SAY THEY WILL DO IT BUT DOING IT ITSELF IS A COMPLETELY DIFFERENT — BECAUSE YOU ARE DOING SOMETHING IS AN ENTIRELY DIFFERENT SUBJECT — NO —"

I broke in on her thoughts and suggested that she could explain this proverb with another one. "YES" she agreed "BUT I DON'T KNOW WHAT IT IS." I began "Actions speak" and D.O. finished "LOUDER THAN WORDS. O.K. CUT. STOP THE TAPE!"

> I HATED THE TAPE RECORDER, I DON'T KNOW WHY. AND AS FOR EXPLAINING PROVERBS, MANY WERE THE DAYS I REMEMBER SAYING "I DON'T LIKE PROVERBS AND DID NOT LIKE EXPLAINING THEM IN SCHOOL!"

Her life was barely her own – for a reason: toward as much speech and muscle progress as possible; toward independence,

Chapter II — By the end of one week

toward a different way of living with satisfactions and joys despite any residual handicaps. Don't give up, keep pushing; keep trying. And always the repeated compliments by us all, the recognition of her effort and of each little but mammoth successful step. Ever onward. And, sometimes, those extra niceties.

> ON THANKSGIVING MORNING MY DAUGHTERS AND HUSBAND BATHED ME AND WASHED MY HAIR. I WAS CLEAN FROM "STEM TO STERN." YES, OF COURSE I WASHED DAILY, BUT THIS PAMPERING WAS LOVELY.

Sessions with the physical therapist were intense: electrical stimulation was used to keep muscles from further atrophy and to stimulate barely functioning nerves. "Feel it, think, and see if you can do the same thing by yourself." This technique required tremendous concentration; beads of sweat dotted D.O.'s face. And, what screams of joy when she was able to cock her right wrist up one-sixteenth of an inch! "Go, Keep Trying, You've Got It!!" Over. And Over. And Over.

Each week new exercises were added. With so much being accomplished at home, speech sessions were cut to once a week with the therapist and physical therapy at the office was reduced to twice a week. Less driving, more responsibility to do everything at home. And, frequent telephone consultations by me with the specialists as some items-to-be-done worked and some didn't.

There was the day when D.O. was to try deep knee bends. I was advised: "Have her back to the wall in the hall; you stand in front of her with your arms extended, your hands under her armpits so that you can support her if her knees give way and she starts to fall." She started down; her knees <u>did</u> collapse --- My first weight-bearing experience in this position – and we both ended up on the floor. My terror: was she all right? Her incredulity! What to do, quick? Laugh – we both laughed hysterically, tears rolling. "Well" I said, "There you are – and you've got to figure out how to get up!" Challenge met, eventually, as we helped each other up. Sweat of panic wiped from my brow, sweat of relief and exhaustion from hers.

"Coffee?"

"YES!"

Time tried to keep pace with her progress.

Chapter III

FRUSTRATIONS: CHORES – CHRISTMAS – PLACES – ASSUMPTIONS

After her stroke, D.O.'s two grown daughters had moved back into the house. Each held jobs and tried to keep the household running smoothly: cooking, laundry, shopping, etc. What support they were, encouraging, loving. D.O. felt guilty, however, about them living at home.

> IT'S NOT NORMAL FOR GROWN CHILDREN TO BE AT HOME. THEY HAD BEEN ON THEIR OWN, AND REALLY SHOULD BE. I LOVED HAVING THEM HERE, BUT I DIDN'T WANT THEM TO FEEL THEY HAD TO STAY BECAUSE OF ME.

But the houseful added to her frustrations:

> EVERYTHING WAS FRUSTRATING – DISHES PUT BACK IN THE WRONG PLACES, THINGS NOT DONE AROUND THE HOUSE THE WAY I USED TO DO THEM. BUT I TRIED NOT TO SAY A WORD ABOUT ALL THIS BECAUSE I KNEW EVERYONE WAS JUST TRYING TO HELP. AND I KNEW THAT WHEN I GOT BETTER I WOULD BE ABLE TO COPE WITH IT ALL. EVERY ONCE IN A WHILE, THOUGH, I WOULD SCREAM – SOMETIMES OUT LOUD!
>
> MORE FRUSTRATIONS WITH YOU, STEVIE, HERE EVERY DAY? I REALLY DON'T THINK SO.... COME

> TO THINK OF IT, YOU WERE HERE WHEN I WOKE UP AND YOU LEFT WHEN MY HUSBAND OR CHILDREN GOT HOME FROM WORK. YES, THERE WERE LOADS OF FRUSTRATIONS: TRYING TO TALK, TRYING TO EXERCISE, TRYING TO WALK – AND YOU MADE ME DO THESE EVEN WHEN I WAS EXHAUSTED. NEVERTHELESS, IN MY MIND THE FRUSTRATIONS WEREN'T YOUR OR ANYONE ELSE'S FAULT.

It was hard for her to put herself first, to concentrate on herself and the things she had to do. The years of giving to her family and friends, of doing for others, made self-focus difficult. Further, as wife and mother, thoughts of family concerns were seldom absent.

Whenever she was alone, it was standard procedure for her husband and children to advise her of their expected time of return. If plans changed, they telephoned with revised schedules. This routine made children who had been on their own return to a pattern of childhood; but, by and large, they adhered to this system. And, whenever I discovered D.O.'s exhaustion in the morning and heard that she had been awake until the wee hours (one or the other had forgotten to call) I chastised the "offender." She did not need this added apprehension or resultant tiredness.

It was almost Christmas. Her son returned from college; he had not seen his mother since her stroke three-and-a-half months ago. She talked to me about him and how she didn't

Chapter III — *Frustrations: Chores - Christmas - Places - Assumptions*

want him to feel hampered or tied down by her present condition; he had his own life to lead. A few days later I overheard her slowly and gently trying to repeat these thoughts to him. I marveled at her strength – and quickly played ball outside with the dogs.

I encouraged her to participate in normal activities of the season, and insisted we go Christmas shopping. We spent an hour in one store, looking; she was unable to make those decisions of what to buy for whom.

> I WAS SCARED TO DEATH ABOUT CHRISTMAS: I DIDN'T THINK I COULD COPE WITH IT. THE FAMILY GOT A CHRISTMAS CATALOGUE AND MADE THE DECISIONS OF WHO GOT WHAT. YOU TOOK ME TO THAT ONE STORE, AND I BOUGHT ONE PRESENT – AN ASHTRAY FOR MY DAUGHTER – BUT I DIDN'T KNOW HOW TO WRAP IT WITH MY LEFT HAND SO I DIDN'T EVEN GIVE IT TO HER.
>
> THAT FIRST CHRISTMAS I WAS DYING TO TELL THE CHILDREN WHAT TO DO WITH SCALLOPED OYSTERS, BUT I COULD NOT DESCRIBE THE PROCEDURE. THE CHILDREN DID THE BEST THEY COULD, AND THE OYSTERS WEREN'T BAD…BUT THEY WEREN'T AS GOOD AS WHEN I COOKED THEM!

Two days before Christmas as we finished a set of exercises she asked me if she could have ten minutes. (Meaning "Can't I have ten minutes off without you insisting on another project?") "Yes, Ma'am." Piece by piece she took the greenery her son had left in the dining room and decorated the living room mantelpiece by herself. Success! It took her forty-five minutes. I was elated that she was beginning to do things she had done before her stroke, that she was starting to have that interest and impetus awakened. "Lovely."

> ON CHRISTMAS DAY I WENT TO THE NURSING HOME WITH MY FAMILY TO SEE MY MOTHER. IT UNDID ME: SHE HAD HAD A SEVERE STROKE, AND I KNEW THAT SHE, TOO, WAS IN BAD SHAPE. SEEING HER REALLY UPSET ME: I LEFT QUICKLY AND WENT TO THE CAR AND SOBBED.

In order to understand some of her problems, I practiced doing things at home with just my left hand. I was a near-failure at the simplest of tasks, and soon realized the importance of teeth as a partial substitute for my right hand. Even so, there were still many times when I could not open things easily or at all (small boxes, plastic containers of food, anything which was wrapped with string). I gave D.O. a pair of left-handed scissors for Christmas – a mirror of right-handed scissors which, I found, did not work on a left hand. These scissors became one of the most useful tools for her, and many were the days when I would have to search for them: she used them in the kitchen, bedroom, and living room – all over the house.

Each day I told the family of her accomplishments and activities. They, in turn, told me of evening happenings, positive

Chapter III — Frustrations: Chores - Christmas - Places - Assumptions

and negative. Try as we did to keep each other informed, there were still gaps in communication which, for me, produced their own particular frustrations. I became angry at what I interpreted as a lack in sensitivity, or at what I considered undue demands made on D.O. by one or another of the family.

One daughter complained that D.O. didn't take any interest in helping to get dinner, and that she usually went to bed right afterwards. I explained the routine her mother and I had during the day – the urging, coaxing to physical and mental activities, and her mother's real exhaustion in the evening. Further, we all had to learn that it took <u>ten times the brain energy now for her mother to do anything</u> – a hard fact to remember and to adjust to.

Her husband, too, upset me when home from work; he wanted to see what his wife had learned to do that day. She and I would be back on the floor <u>again</u>, trying to repeat a motion under duress and with tears of fatigue and frustration (sometimes she could repeat the motion, sometimes not). I did not challenge his demands in front of her. But when she left the room, I told him, too, of the tremendous effort she had already expended during the day and how, in my opinion, she needed his understanding, not his demands.

He was tough. He had his own struggles years before with bulbar polio; he said that it took him ten years of work to regain the use of various swallowing and pulmonary functions. "She can do it if she works hard enough." I could not argue against this line of thought. I tried to understand and be aware of the anguish he must have, at the traumatic alterations of his life, too. His "demands," I reminded myself, were another form of support: he cared, and was not willing to let D.O. give up. This motivation was constant; I treaded lightly.

The rehabilitation process was hard for everyone. Small things usually taken for granted in daily living assumed different proportions and seemed more important now – and were often the cause of friction because, in a sense, they <u>were</u> more important. But as long as we were all in agreement on basic aims and goals (we were) I smoothed over these occasional times of tension (mine, or theirs) and did not tell D.O. of these incidences.

One day off for Christmas and back to work. D.O. continued to try writing with her left hand.

> I STARTED TO WRITE WITH MY LEFT HAND IN THE REHABILITATION HOSPITAL. THE NURSES WERE SURPRISED AT HOW WELL I DID AND ASKED ME IF I WAS NORMALLY LEFT-HANDED!

It was slow. Worse, she could not always spell the word she had finally chosen to write. This was a real blow for this woman of above-average intelligence to whom writing had been second nature.

> IN WRITING A LETTER I WOULD SAY TO MYSELF "I HAD A WONDERFUL TIME" – BUT I HONESTLY DID NOT KNOW WHAT LETTER THE WORDS STARTED WITH, THAT WAS THE REAL PROBLEM. BOOKS

Chapter III — Frustrations: Chores - Christmas - Places - Assumptions

AND DICTIONARIES DID NOT HELP. THE ONLY THING THAT SAVED ME, AS WHEN TRYING TO SPELL "WONDERFUL," WAS TO THINK OF ALL THE WORDS I KNEW WHICH SOUNDED THE SAME TO BEGIN WITH. ONCE I GOT THE FIRST COUPLE OF LETTERS, I COULD SEE THE REST OF THE WORD IN MY HEAD AND THEN WRITE IT. I HAD AN AWFUL TIME WITH MY SPELLING, AND STILL DO.

THERE WAS ANOTHER PROBLEM, TOO: SOMETIMES I WROTE A SYNONYM FOR THE WORD I WAS THINKING – AS "MARVELOUS" INSTEAD OF "WONDERFUL," I DID NOT ALWAYS REALIZE WHAT I HAD DONE. AS A MATTER OF FACT, I STILL DO THIS, TOO.

Two short sentences were the maximum possible at one time. She did not like to be corrected. Nor was I always comfortable, correcting her: this was not "normal adult behavior." But this position of "teacher" was an integral part of the program, and I tried to be more disciplined in my speaking patterns, too. Both of us were learning.

I did not always anticipate the coming directions of the specialists. In most cases, these were given during therapy, in front of D.O. There could be no misunderstanding then – and no chance for either of us to resist the idea of having to do a particularly difficult exercise or procedure.

"Tomorrow you must pry open the fingers of her right hand, one by one, and work each joint," said the physical therapist.

Shivers ran down my back: I knew the pain would be horrendous. It must be done. Before leaving that afternoon, D.O. and I talked about it: I told her that I was not looking forward to doing this, and that I knew she was not eager for it, either. However, we had no choice – so let's get it done first thing in the morning. She agreed. I slept little that night.

When I arrived the next morning, she was still in bed. Putting cold packs on her right hand and arm, we went through the standard question and answer period of last evening's activities, and I did the usual stretching exercises with her right leg. We had a cup of coffee. About 8:30 I asked if she was ready. "YUP." No more was said as I removed the cold packs and unbent her right arm until it was straight on the bed. As gently as possible, literally holding my breath, I took her locked-fist right hand with my left. I did not look at her face as I wiggled the right forefinger of my right hand into the tight circle of her fingers; they locked onto mine – I was surprised a the pressure required to straighten them out. I needed two hands – one to hold her right hand and forearm on the bed (otherwise it would bend with spasticity across her chest), and the other to pry, straighten and move all her fingers. Even with the partial numbness from the cold packs, the pain she experienced was intense; she gripped the covers with her left hand, her left leg bent up, the tears welled over, and she moaned with each pressure on her joints. It was one of the most unpleasant tasks I have ever had to perform.

Chapter III — Frustrations: Chores - Christmas - Places - Assumptions

Five minutes seemed like an hour before I released her fingers which then resumed a fist position. Only then did I look directly at her face and, giving her some Kleenex, thanked her for having let me do this painful exercise.

> WE HAD A JOB TO DO, YOU AND I. THERE WAS NEVER ANY QUESTION ABOUT IT HAVING TO BE DONE. YOU KNOW, THE SAYING GOES "NO PAIN, NO GAIN." I ACTUALLY THINK YOU WERE MORE NERVOUS ABOUT FORCING MY FINGERS OPEN THAN I WAS: I KNEW IT WOULD HURT, BUT I ALSO KNEW THAT IT WOULDN'T LAST LONG, AND THAT IF MY FINGERS WERE EVER TO BE RELAXED AND STRAIGHT, WE HAD TO DO SOMETHING ABOUT THEM RIGHT THEN. STEVIE, IF THE ROLES HAD BEEN REVERSED, YOU WOULD HAVE FELT THE SAME WAY.

The finger-stretching continued each day, once a day, for several weeks. Ever so gradually, the pain subsided and spasticity lessened: her right hand was no longer a locked fist! While doing this procedure, however, a new obstacle came into focus: there seemed to be a connection, hand/shoulder, so that when working with her right hand, spasms of pain were triggered in the right shoulder area also. Another thing to be dealt with.

A learning situation for all: little things took on proportions larger than normal. A "cold" was a real stop, period; blisters on D.O.'s right foot could become infected and stop all gait training, the purposeful re-learning of patterns of walking: Or, the power just developing in various muscle groups could easily regress with lack of continued work. Nothing was static.

Buildings we visited regularly for speech and physical therapy had their own individual potential hazards. At one, the outside double door was too heavy for D.O. to open and keep her balance at the same time. I held my breath wondering if someone would be coming out just as we were trying to go in (sometimes this did happen, with embarrassment on all sides). The other office, in a large hospital on the second floor, posed similar but different hazards: the bank of elevators, so convenient, was at the same time an unusual challenge for D.O. as we waited right next to the one we believed would open first. We were never the only ones waiting, nor did the elevators arrive empty. As a door opened, people pushed – coming out, going in. I learned to stand two feet behind her in case she was inadvertently pushed from behind, and tried to catch the eyes of those getting off in a silent plea to them to be aware of her and go around her. Sometimes we were lucky: another passenger would push the "Hold Open" button for the doors; or sometimes I found myself a physical barrier to their closure.

Shortly after Christmas as we approached the hospital she announced that we would walk up the stairs, that she had done this with her son the day before! It was a long marble staircase, with railings on either side. As we started up, she holding the rail on the left side, I realized another problem: D.O. and I were going up on the left side and would come down on the left,

Chapter III — *Frustrations: Chores - Christmas - Places - Assumptions*

against normal traffic flow. And she was slow, each step pre-thought – what muscles work what so that she could bend her right knee and then straighten it. We stopped in the middle of the flight to look around. Perhaps because her progress up or down was so slow, people did see us ahead of time and circled around us. After the first successful venture, we stopped using the elevator.

Between all the various schedules, appointments with physicians were squeezed in. The day came when we had to see yet another specialist to check on D.O.'s shoulder, now more painful and swollen. It was her first visit to this physician's office. I read aloud the questions which needed to be filled in on standard forms, and D.O. told me what to write. It was a tedious procedure, for whenever there was real pressure to perform (in this case, to give date of birth, address, telephone number, medical history, etc.) D.O. had the most difficulty speaking. I had to laugh at the situation, it was ludicrous: I could read and write quickly, but only she knew the answers. "This is ridiculous," I told her, "they can get all this medical information from your own doctor!" I returned the form, half-completed.

My blood pressure soared whenever anyone anywhere assumed because of her gait or slow speech that D.O. could not understand what was being said or going on around her; it happened here. "Please get her undressed" attacked my sensibilities. After the examination, the physician told <u>me</u> that D.O. should continue with the exercise program, there was no problem. I could barely talk. I told D.O. later of my intense reaction as a form of apology for my fellow man; she lectured me: it had happened so often before, she said she was used to it. I said I would always get angry; she suggested that I was overreacting.

Each day had its ups and downs and I must smooth, react, and bend to those whims of fancy or frustration, all the while remembering the goal of independence and function and the necessary immediate steps toward those ends. D.O. had trouble with names, often using the dog's name instead of mine. I answered whenever she called – and sometimes she was puzzled how come I answered when she had called the dog? (I didn't explain…"My hearing is off" I said lamely.) I interceded and intercepted those endless phone calls of charity or sales, but she talked now to friends whenever it was convenient. I learned to add a little cold water to cups of coffee so visitors would not prolong visits, or she unduly delay working.

I wore many hats and learned to switch them quickly. I had to be aware of moods and changes, of possible physical hazards in case she should fall; or little (but big) things she was trying to do by herself. I always reacted with a nod or a silent smile (if not outright glee): she saw, she knew, she cared what I thought regarding her efforts (or her "cheats").

She <u>was</u> starting to cheat. Certain phrases were in use now to end the necessity for further speech effort on her part: "beats me" – "have it your way" – "I don't know about the common market" (she did!). I implored: "Sentences, please,

Chapter III — *Frustrations: Chores - Christmas - Places - Assumptions*

madam – and knock off those pat answers!" Resignation; regroup. Try again.

Occasionally we tried French, that language of college days. The speech therapist was startled once when D.O. answered a question in French; I interpreted (D.O. answered correctly): another joke between us.

New Year's Eve, a regular workday. In the afternoon, D.O. fought, deciding that no way was she going onto the floor <u>again</u> for exercises. "NO!" Battle/confrontation. Gentle teasing, prodding, poking – even threats of ice cubes – had no effect. What to do? I retreated to a bedroom. "I'll be there if you want me." Silence. Thoughts raced as I lay down: supposing she decided "To hell with it all, I'm not going to do anything anymore…" would I spend the next two hours here in the bedroom, then leave, for good? Or, was she just asserting her independence, indicating "THIS IS MY LIFE, I AM IN CHARGE?" Twenty minutes later I heard her approach (the brace sometimes squeaked). I assumed the "pelvic tilt" position (one of her exercises) and, as she appeared with a slightly guilty little-girl look, I said "Heavens, I don't see <u>how</u> you can hold this position and breathe at the same time!" She broke into laughter, it was contagious; all was well. "C'MON" she ordered, and we went back to the living room floor for exercises. As I left for home, she looked up: "DO YOU STILL LOVE ME?" "Yeah, sometimes. Happy 1975 and I'll see you bright and early in two days."

Chapter IV

GAMES AND NON-GAMES

We played games constantly. Only they were not always fun.

Kick the drawer shut with your right leg;

Shake hands; c'mon, squeeze <u>hard</u>;

Indian-wrestle;

Catch the silly ball;

What's the word for _____?

Name six synonyms for _____;

Tell me what you did last evening, in sequence, in sentences.

Threats of ice cubes or tickling occasionally carried out. Or when, on her back on the floor, and I was preparing to resist the straightening of her right leg, D.O.'s game of straightening her leg before I was balanced, sending me reeling backwards, screeching. Anything to goad, to push.

All leg exercises – originally assisted, lifted, by me – were now done against resistance, strength against strength, another kind of non-game. She practiced walking daily, sometimes checking herself in a mirror at the end of the hall in her house. At the physical therapist's one morning, D.O.'s gait was the focus of attention as the therapist watched her from behind, and I walked backwards, in front of D.O., to watch what she was doing from that angle. Laughter erupted as I walked backwards right into another patient – a predicament D.O. had anticipated and had allowed to happen. Humor, that special ingredient without which the hours would have been so tedious.

The family had always played table-top games, and now was no exception. Checkers were regularly played by D.O. and her husband: after Christmas, a new three-dimensional kind at which she quickly became expert. This was soon followed by Scrabble; I was hard put to equal, much less beat her scores. Games were fun, all participated equally – and they were yet another form of stimulation.

One day it hit me: D.O. could not give directions. For weeks I had assumed I was "dumb," could not find things she wanted or do something she asked. No wonder: she could not say specifically where things were or how to do something. I told the speech therapist. She suggested this problem be added to the agenda, that drills be made up to correct it. Again it was stressed how valuable it was to have someone in the home to see and hear the problems of everyday functioning which the specialists missed in office visits.

We started with "Where is?" organizing thoughts from the general (a room) to the particular part of the room (side) to the specific piece of furniture, to the exact drawer and which side of the drawer. (This was good for memory, too.) It was hard. I wrote what D.O. said, or sometimes we used the tape recorder (she, unwillingly). I proceeded to follow the directions, literally. At first, I found myself looking for her glasses in the sock drawer, or the tea kettle in the bathroom. Besides doing this as an exercise, it became standard operating procedure for anything she wanted, even if I already knew its location. This was really "nitpicking"; sometimes she could not take it: "Never mind, I'll get it myself!"

> TO THIS DAY I CAN STILL PICTURE WHERE SOMETHING IS AND DESCRIBE ITS WHEREABOUTS BECAUSE YOU DRILLED AND DRILLED AND DRILLED ME.

Repetition over and over; nag, scold, plead, scream, and swear. Each day's schedule left little time with nothing to do as new exercises piled on old, physical and verbal.

A Typical Day's Schedule Four Months After Her Stroke

8:00 a.m.	I arrive. Coffee, stretching right leg, structured speech.
8:30	All dressed; make bed; pick up & hang up clothes; wash stockings.
9:00	Lying on bed, cold packs applied to right hand and shoulder
9:05	Start speech drills, verbs.
9:20	Remove cold packs; exercise right hand, fingers, and wrist.

I DID IT! (You did it!!)

9:50	Coffee, juice, chat
10:00	Read aloud.
10:15	Get ready to go and leave for speech therapy.
11:00	Speech Therapy
Noon	Back to car.
12:30	Home; fix lunch.
1:00 p.m.	By yourself time; nap.
1:35	Speech drills; directions; cold packs again.
1:50	Exercises: fingers, hand, right shoulder and arm.
2:30	Ride stationary bicycle.
3:00	Tea time; relax.
3:10	Analyze article for speech; synonyms.
3:30	To kitchen counter; right hand and child's blocks: hold, release.
4:05	Cold packs again; work on verbs again.
4:30	Exercises: right hand; arm; shoulder. On floor: both legs in, out, up and down; on stomach same exercises. Sit-ups.
5:10	Get up from floor unassisted
5:15	Coffee; chat of today's pluses and tomorrow's "need to do's."
5:30	I leave.

Chapter IV — *Games and non-games*

Things normally not my business became so: she was an individual within the framework of home and family, community and world. It was a shock, however, when I was asked by the specialists to inquire about sex. D.O.'s and my backgrounds did not foster such discussion; one did not talk on this subject. I protested to the specialists to no avail; they were insistent.

With shuffling feet and stumbling words I talked first to her husband: "I don't know what your 'sex life' was before D.O.'s stroke, but I need to know whether what you were doing or were not doing before you are doing or not doing today?" Idiotic that I could not be more specific. Even so, he was quick to realize the implications, and answered that yes they did, yes they are, and yes they each have problems but yes they are working them out. Later that day while driving home from the therapist's I told D.O. to look out the window, that I had been directed to ask her some questions which were really not my business but, in a way, they were. The questions were repeated. I dared not look at her. She was gentle with her answers, corroborating what her husband had said. I emphasized to them both what they already knew: that each partner still needed to be needed, that sex was an integral part of their relationship, and that there were solutions to any problems of response or technique.

That evening I related the answers to the specialists. And while still protesting at my having had to ask them about sex, the physical therapist enlarged my perspective: "If you can talk about sex, with each of them separately, you can talk about anything." Obvious, but not so obvious. I lit another cigarette.

> WHEN I FIRST MET YOU SEVERAL YEARS AGO I REMEMBER BUMMING CIGARETTES WHENEVER MY FAMILY WASN'T LOOKING. MY HUSBAND AND I WERE TRYING TO STOP THEN: I WASN'T VERY SUCCESSFUL. WHEN I HAD MY STROKE I WAS SO SICK AND SO SCARED THAT I GAVE IT UP VOLUNTARILY. AND, ONCE I HAD GONE WITHOUT THEM FOR 10 DAYS IN THE INTENSIVE CARE UNIT, I WAS SCARED TO START SMOKING AGAIN. FOR THE FIRST YEAR, THOUGH, WHENEVER I SAW MY BRAND OF CIGARETTES LYING AROUND, I WOULD GET ONE OUT AND RAISE IT TO MY LIPS AND THEN THINK "WHAT THE...I DON'T SMOKE!" IT WAS A HABIT, BUT I DON'T REALLY MISS IT.

Humor, more than once the saving grace of a situation. She was stopped at the check-out counter of the grocery store; someone assumed from her walk that she had a cast on her leg, and being in Colorado in winter had had a skiing accident. D.O. never batted the proverbial eye: "I'm getting better!" As we left, she laughed; I laughed with her --- and bled a little on the inside: oh, that it were that simple. Damn.

We advanced to: "Tell me, in sequence, how to make coffee." She: "IF YOU DON'T KNOW HOW, I WON'T WASTE IT ON YOU ANYMORE!" "C'mon," I pleaded, "be serious! Instead, tell me how to make an old fashioned...and if you don't tell me sequentially, there won't be any tonight!" D.O. did not miss a verbal step!

Chapter IV — Games and non-games

DID YOU MIND HAVING SOUP FOR LUNCH ALMOST EVERY DAY? FOR SIX MONTHS AFTER MY STROKE NOTHING TASTED GOOD AND SO WHEN YOU INSISTED I MAKE THE LUNCH I JUST OPENED A CAN OF SOUP. FURTHERMORE, I WAS NOT ABOUT TO TRY TO SPREAD THE BREAD FOR SANDWICHES WITH ONLY MY LEFT HAND. EVEN TODAY I DON'T ESPECIALLY LIKE TO MAKE SANDWICHES, BUT I <u>CAN</u> MAKE THEM NOW.

Moods and activities precluded boredom as each day brought different challenges. And whenever the roads were really icy, therapy in town was cancelled and it was rather like a school holiday – with a difference: although we might light a fire and have a more relaxed day, still, hours were spent on regular strengthening and stretching exercises and on purposeful speech drills. But what fun if the ice melted later in the day and we went shopping or out for lunch or to visit a friend.

Stretching exercises for D.O.'s right arm were even more painful; it had to be ranged and raised in all positions. She could not do this herself; I had to do it for her. The first time I practiced raising D.O.'s right arm at the therapist's I experienced all the anguish of knowing the pain, of seeing my friend brace herself and then sob.

IS IT GOING TO BE LIKE THIS FOREVER?

"No way," I answered, and reminded her of the awful involuntary shoulder spasms which had now almost disappeared, e.g. this, too, will pass. The next few weeks were difficult with arm-stretching twice a day. And not once did she try to avoid having it done.

> GET TO IT. LET'S FINISH UP SO YOU WILL GO HOME!

Many were the days when I was an emotional wreck by the time I went home. Despite naps snuck in when D.O. was resting, I was exhausted – physically, mentally and emotionally.

There were times when she did not want to get up and said so; or when she announced that she was going to sit in a chair all day, period. Each occurrence demanded a different response; I mentally rearranged schedules and weighed the advantages of "pushing" or not pushing. Guilt came easily to D.O. as she would apologize for "not doing very well today." I showed her that it was normal for her to be sick of all she had to do, that it was normal to want to sit – but that no way would any of us let her sit too long: <u>that was not an on-going option!</u>

> I AM IMPATIENT. I WANT TO BE WELL, <u>NOW</u>. FURTHER, I HAD THOSE PERIODS OF BEING TIRED – TIRED OF ALWAYS PUSHING, EXERCISING: TIRED OF BEING. BUT I KNEW THEN AS I KNOW NOW THAT I HAVE NO CHOICE BUT TO KEEP WORKING, THAT THIS IS THE ONLY WAY I'LL BE ABLE TO LEARN TO WALK MORE NORMALLY, THE ONLY WAY I CAN LEARN TO MAKE MY RIGHT HAND FUNCTION OR MY SPEECH BETTER.

Chapter IV — *Games and non-games*

Rehabilitation – the restoration to a state of health and useful activity through training, therapy and guidance – was (and is) an agonizingly slow process. Just because things were once accomplished did not mean that they would be again when severe brain damage had occurred. Although brain cells do not regenerate, still there is an infinite number of cells which are not normally trained or in use, and untold millions of nerve connections. The rehabilitation process harnessed every opportunity possible to foster the development of abilities, the functioning of these cells to their maximum potential. The extent to which these efforts would succeed was unpredictable.

D.O.'s impatience was not bizarre. We all learned that results were not, in most instances, instantaneous, that patience and repetition were ongoing necessities. But each little step forward was a mammoth achievement resulting in indescribable joy for her and for all of us.

Work continued with added perspectives: she was afraid of falling, and yet might someday do so when no one was around. She had to be able to get up from the floor by herself and without the aid of tables or sofas; these supports might not always be available.

After floor exercises late one afternoon I insisted that she try to get up alone. She was terrified, shaking, and determined to edge her way over to a table for help, sliding on her knees. I blocked her way. Her daughters came home from work to find us on the floor, and I explained the situation. "Don't be stubborn, Mom." "I'LL FIRE YOU," D.O. said. I held my breath. She was quite serious. But, right now, she had to get off her knees! "I know you may fire me," I answered. "But, right now, Get Up!" She was near tears. I finally held her left arm, and she got up and went directly into the kitchen. The next morning the family told me of her real anger, how she had telephoned me that night (I was out). I trod carefully until the afternoon when we talked about it. D.O. recognized the logic of self-care, and capitulated, grimly agreeing to practice getting up several times each day with me by her side until she could master the technique and feel safer.

One late wintry afternoon we were all in the living room: D.O., her husband and daughters, and her son who had not yet returned to college. I was on the floor near the fire as conversation was light about the day's activities. Suddenly, the talk was serious: her husband demanded that D.O. set goals for herself, now, aloud. The room was silent; my stomach knotted: why now? Why this pressure to remember, to set goals which no one knows the possibility of attainment? Why, in front of the children? Why, in front of me? D.O. stared at the brightly burning fire as she searched for the words and answers, her speech painfully slow, broken by sobs. After what seemed an eternity, she finally named two goals: talking better, and throwing pottery again. Her husband hammered home the rationale that if she worked hard, she could accomplish whatever she realistically set out to do – but that she had to work hard, every day.

Chapter IV — *Games and non-games*

The rest of us were quiet. I was especially so, stifling those emotions of sorrow at this situation and anger at her husband. I left shortly thereafter, wishing I could "boil him in oil." It was only many weeks later that I glimpsed again his means of motivation, that I realized his own questions as he himself pondered his wife's future of uncertainties.

Such episodes, rare as they were, upset my equilibrium. I talked to the specialists, as much to keep them abreast of things happening in the home as to gain insights from their individual experiences. The stories they told of disillusionment, despair and family rupture did much to dispel my anguish. They assured me all the ingredients for progress were present in D.O.'s rehabilitation. It was obvious that each family member cared and provided further motivation for her. That I saw and heard things to which the specialists were not privy in office visits enlarged our understanding of this one situation and aided us all in strategies for this particular patient. They reminded me that we should all be aware of family coping patterns, and that we could not force changes in these patterns which had been formed over the years. How comforting it was for me to be able to talk with them!

Primarily because of these perspectives I gradually accepted the instances of family pressure which occurred regularly. These were deliberate attempts to will D.O. into action, to help her develop a self image based even now on her worth as a human being, as a wife and mother. Her husband was relentless – and his influence of incalculable benefit.

There was a new movie in town, "The Little Prince." D.O. remembered the story from childhood, and so on a cold gray afternoon we condensed homework and exercises in order to see it. I was not at all sure whether she would be able to follow the movie's pace of speech and images, but I hoped that with her familiarity of the subject she would not be overwhelmed by frustration. And it was something we had not done or tried before.

There was a line for tickets at the theater, and I winced, knowing how easily she became cold. Braving onlookers' curious glances, we went inside where I asked and received permission for D.O. to wait while I took my turn in the line outside. We sat on the aisle and indulged in popcorn and soda like everyone else. And like everyone else, both of us were soon engrossed in the unfolding story – I in perceiving her visual and auditory reception and comprehension and she <u>with the movie</u>! In the lobby, while leaving the theater, she suddenly called "STOP!" She had contracted a severe spasm in her right shoulder. There was nothing I could do except steer her to a bench where we sat for a few minutes until the pain became less jabbing. Overall, though, it was a successful outing. D.O. enjoyed the interruption of routine <u>and</u> the movie.

It was midwinter. Her husband had to go on a short business trip to Florida in a few weeks. "CAN I GO?" D.O. asked. All agreed it would be good, she needed a break. But first, preparation for going on the trip, swimming with the therapist on one side, and I the other: good for exercise in the water as

Chapter IV   —   *Games and non-games*

well as showing her that she was "water-safe." Her water temperature tolerance too, had changed: pools we used had to be much warmer than normal.

Once again, the unexpected. A pool we had been in one morning was later found to be contaminated. The physical therapist called us that afternoon and required self-examination, both of us, immediately, with any open scratches or blisters to be reported back to her (there were none). Bathe in tincture of green soap followed by an alcohol rub. Both of us. Now. It was serious, it was funny, it was hilarious as imaginations took hold and we swatted non-existent bugs. The situation was…unusual! It enhanced bonds.

The day before departure for Florida arrived. D.O. was shown how to do various stretching exercises by herself and was on her own to do them while away. Packing was another adjustment (how to fold and pack with her left hand?) The skies darkened; it started to snow. "Maybe the planes will be grounded tomorrow" I teased. "<u>I AM GOING NO MATTER WHAT. I'LL…TAKE A …BUS IF I HAVE TO</u>!" she retorted. The next day dawned clear and they were off. I was anxious that all should go well.

She came home tanned, "wide-eyed and bushy-tailed" and not eager to return to the work routine. "YOU CAN GO HOME ANYTIME," she said. "Thanks," I replied, "but I'm NOT leaving!" She was argumentative that first day back. And negative about everything. By mid-afternoon I couldn't resist saying (to no one in particular) "Thank heaven the sun is out – everything else around here has been so glum that it's nice to see the sun!" The message worked: she broke out laughing, and the following days were as usual again.

There was new homework for speech: from now on D.O. was to read aloud fifteen minutes a day and was to take notes while watching the news on T.V. I was instructed to monitor her speech all the time: if there were errors of usage or pronunciation, she was to be stopped and told of the errors (if she had not recognized them in the saying) and should start that sentence all over again. The hope was that with constant monitoring she would eventually be able to automatically self-correct. In the meantime, she had to learn to really hear what she was saying. I was uncomfortable: it was not my nature to nitpick on a constant basis. Further, I knew she would balk at these corrections. The speech therapist explained that it was far better for me to be doing this than the family.

Using a list of words from the dictionary, I sometimes asked D.O. to name synonyms for each word, and to make up appropriate sentences:

Accord:

"THE CHOIR IS IN HARMONY."

Does "accord" have the same meaning as that? Does it have anything to do with music?

"IT DOES TO ME!"

Accumulate:

"I AMASS — O.K., I HOARD — OH, WELL, I ACCUMULATE LOTS OF STUFF."

That's for sure.

"YOU DON'T — YOU DON'T — YOU DO NOT DO SO BAD YOURSELF!"

Accurate:

THE ACCURATE READING IS ZERO.

O.K.

Accursed:

THE ACCURSED SPOT IS NOT COMING OUT.

O.K.

Accused:

COMMIT — COMMIT A CRIME?

No.

OH, WELL, I ACCUSE YOU OF MAKING MONEY WITH ILLEGAL MONEY — NO. I ACCUSE YOU OF MAKING ILLEGAL MONEY.

O.K.

There were times when she refused to say more than one word or short sentence in answer to the usual questions:

What did you do this past weekend?

    THE USUAL.

What?

    I HAVEN'T GOT ANYTHING OF INTEREST.

Did you go out for dinner Friday evening?

    YUP.

Where?

    A NEIGHBOR'S.

What did you have for dinner?

    FOOD!

Did you play bridge?

    YUP.

Who won at bridge?

    I DON'T KNOW.

I thought you kept score?

    I DIDN'T RECORD IT.

Chapter IV — Games and non-games

Where's your husband?

GONE.

Gone? Where?

OHIO.

What's he doing in Ohio?

TALKING BUSINESS!

What can we talk about?

NOTHING.

Period. Laughter – and the tape was turned off, to be saved for a more voluble session.

Spring arrived and with it new realities and frustrations: friends on the tennis courts again, everyday. "You'll be back on the courts any day now," a visitor said. "EACH DAY I'M GETTING BETTER, LITTLE BY LITTLE" D.O. answered. True, but tennis again? I was silent; this is a fast, well-coordinated game for anyone. Today she could not run, walking was still difficult, she could not hold a racket. Bleed inwardly; work onward.

To change the routine further we devised physical activity, games, wherein the same muscle groups would be strengthened in a more functional setting and hopefully a more fun one. Dry-land skiing up and down the hall, ladders for walking between the rungs evenly; rope for jumping (walking) over, hockey stick to hit the plastic ball using both arms; large balls to catch and push away.

> I REALLY DIDN'T LIKE THOSE GAMES, ESPECIALLY THE ONE WHERE WE KICKED A LARGE BALL BACK AND FORTH ON THE FRONT LAWN. AND THEN, TO MAKE IT WORSE, YOU GOT A BUSHEL BASKET AND I WAS SUPPOSED TO KICK THE BALL INTO IT FOR A "GOAL." THERE WAS I, A GROWN WOMAN, KICKING A BALL WITH ANOTHER GROWN WOMAN – I FELT VERY FOOLISH. I KNEW WHY WE DID THOSE GAMES, BUT I REALLY THOUGHT THEM STUPID AND THAT THERE MUST BE OTHER WAYS TO ACCOMPLISH THOSE ENDS.

Physical therapy was more than hours spent at an office, learning and practicing with a therapist. It was almost another world where patients and staff all knew each other and all were genuinely interested in each other's problems and progress. Therapy took place in small rooms, or in a larger one with space for extended walking. No one seemed surprised when D.O. and I arrived once with the large plastic ball and hockey stick. But we were all surprised and pleased as she managed to keep her right hand on the stick and hit the ball down the length of the large room. It stopped near a male patient severely disabled with arthritis. He kicked the ball back to D.O.! It was delightful, it was magnificent, and we all cheered as each of them became completely engrossed, oblivious of onlookers, caught in their own game of chance and determination.

Chapter IV — Games and non-games

Thinking up things for D.O. to do as another form of exercise was challenging. Occasionally, my enthusiasm for the task overshadowed wisdom as my ideas became, for D.O., indignities. Good intentions were not enough as I discovered with mortification one gray spring afternoon. I decided that croquet wickets would be perfect for an exercise to strengthen those muscles which aid in lifting her right knee (as in walking). On the pretext of checking for flowers, we went outside where I had already set up the wickets in a row. My instructions to her were clear; she must walk <u>over</u> the wickets. Her enthusiasm was less than overwhelming and equally clear: she did not want to walk over the wickets. Her son, home from college for spring break, was persuaded to block her path should she try to go back into the house. It was another war of wills. Eventually, she did walk over the wickets, once, then "marched," in silence, back to the house.

I kicked myself for having crossed that fine line of sensitivity. "Coffee?" I asked – and we proceeded to conversation.

Most of our talking now was consciously structured to stimulate thinking and response on as wide a variety of subjects as possible. There was the normal chat of home and family; but, in addition, I initiated discussions at least twice a day on current events, history, anything which would force D.O. to think both practically and in the abstract. Her educational background assured her general knowledge: philosophy, art, music or global politics. She had difficulty defending and explaining a position; when flustered her speech was more faltering and experimental.

I often took opposite viewpoints in order to lengthen the discussion, to make her keep trying to explain her stance. I smiled as I found myself defending a position opposite to what I really thought and wondered if I was "the fool."

Seldom do two or more people agree with each other on everything. Just as there were occasions with D.O. or her family, there were also times of disagreement among one or other of the specialists. These moments were never shared with D.O.; for all intents and purposes we presented a united front.

Whenever cracks appeared in this solidarity, I found myself in the middle, trying to balance the wishes of specialists who sometimes seemed to forget that there was anything else to be done outside of his or her special area of concern with their patient. On the job, I tipped the balance in whichever direction the moment's need seemed to dictate – and occasionally purposefully ignored the list for the day with the conviction that living needed to be done, too. Whenever I told the specialists of these on-the-spot-decisions, they were supportive and enthusiastic – and then reminded me of their own program plans which must be done!

Exercises and cold packs were not forgotten. Late one afternoon when D.O. was telling me to rearrange these packs yet another time and I was whistling away this persnickety procedure, I was suddenly aware of harmony: she was whistling too! "I did not know you could whistle again; how long have you been able to do that?" Smugly, "OH, FOR A

Chapter IV — Games and non-games

LONG TIME! I'VE BEEN PRACTICING!!" (Music to my ears, whistling – and practicing.)

As speaking got easier and her normal reticence to discuss feelings became less, D.O. spoke about having had a stroke and her immediate reactions in the hospital:

> I WAS IN A ROOM, SURROUNDED BY DOCTORS. SOMEONE SAID, "MASSIVE STROKE," AND I REMEMBER THINKING I MIGHT DIE. BUT I WASN'T AFRAID. I THOUGHT OF THE CHILDREN, AND HOW THEY WERE GROWN AND DID NOT REALLY NEED ME. I THOUGHT OF MY HUSBAND (she cried now, remembering). AND THEN ANOTHER DOCTOR SAID, "SHE'S ONLY 47, SHE'S TOO YOUNG!" AND I SAID TO MYSELF "I'M TOO YOUNG!" I SUPPOSE THAT WAS MY TURNING POINT, THAT SUBCONSCIOUSLY I BEGAN TO FIGHT TO SURVIVE.
>
> THE DAYS I SPENT IN THE HOSPITAL ARE BLURRED; I WAS NOT ALWAYS FULLY CONSCIOUS. I REMEMBER VISITS FROM MY FAMILY AND A COUPLE OF CLOSE FRIENDS. SOMETIMES I WAS STRAPPED IN A WHEELCHAIR, AND I FELT INDIGNANT AT BEING STRAPPED.
>
> I DON'T KNOW HOW OR WHY I HAD A STROKE; SOMETHING WENT WRONG, OBVIOUSLY. IF IT HAPPENED ONCE, WILL IT HAPPEN AGAIN?

She was learning to talk, figuratively and practically. She was sorting – and evaluating.

Her children commented: her stroke had brought them all closer together. Yes. At the same time, each family member, in his or her own way, was a participant in the on-going support and pressure. All played significant roles, and all adjusted – daily it seemed – as D.O. slowly took back the responsibilities she once had in the home.

She was not content now, to let others keep doing household chores; the laundry, for instance, was <u>her</u> job. She experimented with ways to get the soiled clothes down to the basement – and up again: with as many clean clothes on hangers as possible, she put the hangers in her teeth and brought them up. Baskets were used in all possible fashions; the laundry would be done! It was exhausting, all these trips to the basement, but I dared not let up. "YOU'RE A CRUEL BEAST" she admonished; "I'M TIRED. YOU GO HOME." (Yes, ma'am, after the last set of exercises.)

I was sometimes torn by the demands we all made of her. But each one had its place in the renewal of function and normal living.

> THERE WERE MANY MORNINGS WHEN I WOULD STILL BE IN BED HOPING THE PHONE WOULD RING AND YOU WOULD SAY YOU WERE SICK! IT ONLY HAPPENED TWICE, BUT WHAT A JOY TO HAVE THE HOUSE ALL TO MYSELF AND NOT HAVE YOU NAGGING ME.

Chapter IV — Games and non-games

She was trying to clean out closets and drawers in addition to all the other work. Taping sessions continued on directions for doing things. They had to be precise, and were on a variety of subjects: how to clean out the fireplace; how to do the laundry and set the washing machine dial; how to plant petunias. And, once, it was on "How Do You Cook African Rock Lobster Tails?"

> WOW, DELICACY DELUXE. YOU BROIL THEM. — WELL, GO TO THE KITCHEN AND YOU SEE TWO LOBSTERS IN THE ICEBOX...

I have the neatest mental picture of those beasts crawling around in the icebox!

> OH... (laughing)... THE LOBSTER IS — THE LOBSTERS ARE COOKED. NO, IT'S NOT COOKED BUT IT'S KILLED.

Whole lobsters?

> NO, TAILS, PLURAL. FIRST YOU GET A BIG PAN — - AND — FILL IT WITH WATER. THEN YOU — PICK THE TAILS OUT OF THE ICEBOX, AND THROW IT IN THE BOILING WATER.

Just one?

> NO, MORE THAN ONE, PLURAL. COOK IT, THEM FOR TEN MINUTES. — DRAIN THE WATER. IT'S FINISHED.

It?

YES, THE COOKING!

I thought you said in the beginning that you had to broil them?

I CHANGED MY MIND SUDDENLY!

Suppose one were going to broil them?

I DON'T KNOW; <u>YOU</u> TRY IT!

One day I was accosted by a long-time friend of D.O.'s: what had happened to D.O.'s personality, I was asked, she was not as agreeable as she used to be or as willing to do something suggested. And D.O. was saying "NO" which she had seldom said before her stroke. It was all I could do not to scream "Hallelujah!" I explained that from now on D.O. would have to be able to say "no" without guilt; that often there would be times when she should not do something that was asked of her; that she had to learn to gauge her abilities realistically, her fatigue-factor honestly. And there would be times when she should indicate "no more pushing, I've had it." We discussed the phrase "Knock it off" which D.O. was now using; I praised this development to her friend. I hoped she would understand. Later I related the gist of this conversation to my "patient" and showered her with compliments. She understood better than any of us.

Chapter V

RESPONSIBILITY SHIFTS

Summer arrived and with it the boredom of skis and balls, hockey stick and ladder; D.O. had grimly endured these occupations which now even I deemed foolish; they had served their purpose, but it was time to move on.

Speech therapy ended on a formal basis. She was told that she had gone beyond available texts and must now continue on her own each day. "Keep discussing, practice speaking all the time," the therapist advised. "And, don't forget the writing: try a typewriter. Don't let up. You will continue to improve, but more slowly."

The specialists and I had discussed the possible psychological impact this development might have. We knew that people generally went only so long in an intensive rehabilitation program before doubts about future progress emerged. Feelings of "what's the use?" were to be expected along the way.

> YOU KNOW, I REALLY THOUGHT THAT I WOULD BE TALKING NORMALLY BY THE TIME I FINISHED SPEECH THERAPY. AND THERE I WAS, STILL NOT TALKING WELL – AND I WAS VIRTUALLY DISMISSED FROM CLASS. THE THERAPIST

SHOWED ME COMPARISONS OF TESTS I HAD DONE RIGHT AFTER MY STROKE AND RECENTLY. I WAS, OF COURSE, PLEASED AT THE UPWARD CURVES. BUT I KNEW MY SPEECH WAS NOT ALL BETTER. I GUESS I REALLY STARTED TO WONDER IF IT EVER WOULD BE. I WAS SCARED.

Depression hit. Though predictable, this did not lessen the concern.

Her husband and daughters were out of town when she voiced those fears of "When will I get better?" and despaired at the thought that she might not. Her anxiety level was high, and she wondered whether she would someday have another stroke. I stayed with her until 1 a.m. and was emotionally spent. Once home, I wrote down what I could remember of the evening's conversation.

Everyday I continued to write. It was a good exercise, and enhanced awareness of all the daily activities and nuances. This morning it was difficult: there was so much to cover. At 7 a.m. I called the physical therapist: D.O. had a scheduled appointment with her that day. I related the past evening's depression. Because of the basic honesty and rapport we three had with each other, the therapist and I decided to change the appointment from an active exercise session to a talk session.

Later that morning the three of us were seated around a table in the conference room…one-and-a-half hours of D.O. "letting it all out…"

Chapter V — Responsibility shifts

IT'S BEEN SIX MONTHS SINCE MY STROKE AND I'M STILL NOT ALL WELL.

<u>There</u> it was.

She was told the uselessness of artificial time lines; no way can one predict when specifics will be possible, or even if they ever will be in certain areas. She was told of the belief from observation and experience that when certain doors closed, others opened; that she must make room for other things, see new possibilities. "And look at what progress you have made, from flat on your back and near death, to walking, taking care of yourself and household duties, some social activities with your husband, a trip to Florida, and tremendous strides with your speech. <u>All This</u>!" Prop, support, love, understand, cry, prop again. I took notes (later shown to her husband and given to D.O. as a visual reminder of the discussion). I could not afford to join in the tears right then: I was afraid that if I began, I might not stop easily. The physical therapist noticed my reserve and teased; we all laughed.

D.O. and I left the physical therapist's with a new assignment of ascertaining hurdles around the house: weight and size of kitchen utensils, better ways to move laundry from one floor to the next, convenience of often-used objects. This was a practical project: it gave us something specific to do with immediate results.

The conversation on the way home was a re-hash of the conference. Over and over I echoed the therapist's words of fact, accomplishment and praise. I believed them, and wanted to force D.O. to believe them, too.

During the next few weeks I followed her, literally, around the house. Initially, D.O. was not enthusiastic about changing anything. I took her set of dishes from the second shelf and rearranged the kitchen cupboard so that they were on the first shelf where she could reach them more easily – a simple thing, but for D.O. this turned out to be much more convenient. Next, we went to the hardware store and bought two items: a plastic colander so that she could wash and drain vegetables more easily; and a special jar opener which, attached to the underside of her cupboard, gripped any size lid so that she could turn the jar with her left hand and it would unscrew. We should have thought of these earlier. Her husband, meanwhile, had begun to build a laundry chute; it was now completed so that she did not have to carry the soiled laundry down to the basement.

As I tagged along, wherever she went, looking for more things we could do or manufacture to make chores easier, it was obvious that she resented my shadow. She was normal!

We split hairs over the definitions of "normal" and "well." Her husband and I insisted one evening that she perceive herself as normal and well. "BUT, I'M NOT," she said. "<u>Yes You Are</u>," we countered, "where it matters: in your head (intellectually) and in your heart (emotionally)." We hammered at this; the facts of slow speech or disturbed motor function were not relevant. She was dubious.

Chapter V — Responsibility shifts

Reading aloud and the discussion of articles continued. It was fun when she picked out something we both knew from firsthand experience. So it was when she read a dissertation about the beaches of Hawaii – where they were, how one had to search for them, etc. The article ended with a description of the island of Kauai. I prodded her memory, and asked if she had ever driven the road on Kauai which "goes around to the right, or north?"

> IT'S NORTH AND SOUTH! WE BOTH — I — WE BOTH DROVE IT SOUTH AND NORTH AT THE FINISH.

Picking up her incorrect phrase, I asked her if they had gotten out "at the finish?"

> I — I DON'T KNOW WHAT YOU MEAN.

I quoted her phrase back to her, and only then did she hear what she had said.

> DO YOU MEAN DID WE GET OUT OF THE CAR AT THE END OF THE ROAD? OH. WELL, YES WE GOT OUT AND WALKED AROUND A BIT.

Her visual pace of events was often far ahead of her conversation. In the Hawaii incident, not only had she not heard the "at the finish," but, in her mind, D.O. had quickly relived the journey on that road and was already back at home base before I asked about details in the middle of the story. "Switching gears" I called it – the ability to jump back and forth in time, or the ability to change subjects quickly and be able to follow the conversation; this, too, we worked on.

As more days passed she demonstrated again the determination to be in control of her life. "Games" emerged wherein my natural gullibility reinforced her own one-upmanship; I <u>was</u> "the fool." Another hat was added; I was slow to recognize its addition – or its worth.

One day I told her of my recent efforts to add oil to my car. This time it was <u>she</u> who demanded a sequential order to <u>my</u> story. With a straight face she questioned the color of the oil reservoir cap I have just laboriously explained to the point where, unsure of my own precision, I went to the car, raised the hood, and, with righteous indignation (it <u>was</u> red!) returned to tell her that I was indeed correct – only to find her doubled over in laughter at my gullibility. I took another breath, and rejoiced in her gamesmanship, another reminder of her normalcy and sense of humor, and that it was she who, in the last analysis, was in charge.

Her husband had to work in Florida for nine weeks, and D.O. was going too. What would she do by herself? Pages of exercises were fine-tooth-combed and adjusted for her to do without assistance. We substituted rubber rings, pulleys, walls for resistance. She was shown how to do ranging of her right arm with ropes and left hand assistance; ranging where a limb must be moved in all directions to keep it limber. The pain was much less, and the spasms almost gone. She was beginning to learn

Chapter V — Responsibility shifts

how to "turn off" those involuntary impulses which forced her hand into a fist, or those which did not allow the bending of her right knee at will. She was accomplishing, but it had to be continued daily. It would be her responsibility now, and she had to do everything calmly, coolly, or it would be impossible.

Any fatigue or tension had immediate effects on D.O.: her speech worsened, her gait worsened, and spasticity appeared full force in her right foot and right hand and arm. Sometimes painful, it was obvious when she had a problem. She had to learn to recognize the signs, identify the problem, and communicate about it, then deal with it. At the time, she could not always isolate what it was that was bothering her.

She could pull her right foot up and out; how long had it been, working on just this one motion? Damaged nerves, faint impulses. Work, work, and try again. Don't forget.

Into one suitcase went all the therapy items she must take with her to Florida: ropes, pulleys, weights, and balls. <u>And</u> the notebook with exercise instructions to remind her what she must do each day and how.

> I REMEMBER THINKING IT WOULD BE NICE IF THAT SUITCASE WERE LOST ON THE WAY TO FLORIDA! YOU WERE REALLY FUNNY WHEN I MENTIONED THIS: YOU SAID, SO SERIOUSLY, THAT AT LEAST YOU HAD A COPY OF ALL THE EXERCISES AND WOULD SEND IT TO ME IF NECESSARY! I WAS ONLY TEASING YOU, BUT I

> THINK YOU WERE NERVOUS ABOUT MY GOING AWAY FOR SO LONG AND WHETHER I WOULD REALLY DO ALL THE EXERCISES EACH DAY. ACTUALLY, I WAS ANXIOUS TOO: I DIDN'T KNOW WHETHER I WOULD BE ABLE TO DO ALL THOSE THINGS BY MYSELF. BUT I WAS EAGER TO GO AND BE WITH MY HUSBAND.

I <u>was</u> apprehensive: she was dependent on me a great deal for support, stimulation, and as a cushion to her falls, real and psychological. Further, the dependence was two ways: she was involved in my life, too; she was <u>my</u> confidante, always there to listen as I expounded on the latest family "traumas." We helped each other with our particular experiences and wisdom. I would miss her, but the trip would give her another chance to test her mettle. I suggested she send me a plane ticket if she got into trouble --- "hip-pocket psychology."

One day before departure there was another problem: something was wrong with the shoe on D.O.'s brace.

> EVERY TIME I WALKED, SOMETHING JABBED THE BOTTOM OF MY RIGHT FOOT. THE PHYSICAL THERAPIST WAS OUT OF TOWN SO WE COULDN'T CALL HER. YOU TRIED MY BRACE ON AND WERE HORRIFIED: YOU SAID THE STEEL SHANK IN THE SOLE OF THE SHOE WAS BROKEN.

I took the brace to the shop where it had been originally made and fitted. After explaining the problem, I pleaded: it had to be fixed in 24-hours because of D.O.'s trip. The technician

Chapter V — Responsibility shifts

understood, and the shank was replaced that day. But when I picked it up, I found that he had also changed the sole of the shoe: it was now 1/2 inch thicker! I inquired whether this might not throw off D.O.'s balance with one shoe higher than the other. This had not occurred to him! Another two trips to town, this time with her normal left shoe in hand; a half inch sole was added, another problem solved, and she was ready for Florida the next day.

A one-page letter, typed, came in a week (another first). It had taken her three hours to do, and indicated many meals, evenings out (good), lovely view (O.K.), swimming (excellent) and husband working hard. I visited D.O.'s mother often in the nursing home; she was gradually failing and worried about her daughter. I bolstered her, and in so doing bolstered myself. And a few weeks later I called Florida and was relieved to hear D.O. well; I reported this to all who asked.

> I REALLY LOVED THAT TRIP. IT WAS WARM IN FLORIDA, BUT THERE WAS ALWAYS A BREEZE SO IT WASN'T TOO HOT. WE WERE IN TWO DIFFERENT CONDOMINIUMS THAT SUMMER. AT THE FIRST ONE, I HAD A MAID COME IN TWICE A WEEK; SHE CHANGED THE BED AND CLEANED THE APARTMENT. WHEN WE MOVED TO THE SECOND PLACE, I DID NOT HAVE ANYONE COME IN TO HELP; THIS WAS THE FIRST TIME I HAD HAD TO CHANGE THE KING-SIZED BED BY MYSELF. I DID NOT KNOW WHETHER I COULD DO IT OR NOT...USING ONE HAND. IT WAS A SLOW

PROCESS, BUT I CHANGED IT! IT WAS NO EASY CHORE, BUT I FELT MARVELOUS THAT I HAD ACTUALLY DONE IT.

EACH DAY I WOULD USUALLY MAKE THE BED, THEN GET INTO MY SWIMMING SUIT AND GO TO THE POOL AND SWIM AND LOUNGE A FEW HOURS. THEN I WOULD GO BACK TO THE APARTMENT FOR THE MAIL, WATCH T.V., THEN GET DRESSED AND GO OUTSIDE AGAIN AND WAIT FOR MY HUSBAND TO GET BACK FROM WORK. I DID TYPE A COUPLE OF LETTERS: THEY TOOK FOREVER! AND I READ A BIT.

OCCASIONALLY I WENT OUT WITH OTHER WIVES WHOSE HUSBANDS WERE WORKING WITH MINE: WE WOULD SHOP, OR HAVE LUNCH. ONE TIME FOUR OF US DECIDED TO PICK ORANGES: THREE OF US GOT QUITE A FEW! I WAS NOT VERY GOOD AT THIS BECAUSE THE TERRAIN WAS VERY UNEVEN AND MOST OF THE ORANGES WERE TOO HIGH FOR ME TO REACH, BUT IT WAS FUN.

I HAD NO PROBLEM BEING BY MYSELF A GOOD DEAL. AND EVERY DAY I DID A FEW EXERCISES – AND SOMETIMES GOT MADDER THAN HELL WHEN SOME OF THEM DIDN'T WORK AS THEY WERE SUPPOSED TO, ESPECIALLY THE ARM-STRETCHING ONES: EVEN WITH THE ROPE AND PULLEY TO HELP I COULD NOT DO THOSE

Chapter V — *Responsibility shifts*

EXERCISES AND RANGING. WHEN I CAME HOME, THOUGH, THE THERAPIST WAS VERY PLEASED WITH MY PROGRESS: OBVIOUSLY THE SWIMMING HAD BEEN GOOD FOR ME. AS A MATTER OF FACT, MY HUSBAND SUPERVISED MY EXERCISES IN THE POOL ALMOST EVERY DAY, ESPECIALLY THOSE FOR MY RIGHT LEG.

WE WERE RIGHT ON THE BEACH AND THE VIEW AND SMELLS OF SALT WATER FROM THE BALCONY WERE PLEASANT. SOMETIMES WE WOULD WALK ON THE BEACH. ONE EVENING WE HAD ASKED TWO OTHER COUPLES OVER FOR A SWIM AND DINNER. WE ALL WENT DOWN TO THE BEACH AND WENT INTO THE WATER. ALL OF A SUDDEN A BIG WAVE CAME AND TOOK MY GLASSES, NO KIDDING! LUCKILY, MY HUSBAND WAS ABLE TO RETRIEVE THEM.

WE ATE OUT QUITE A FEW TIMES – AND I EVEN TRIED DANCING AND HAVE A PICTURE TO PROVE IT! ALTOGETHER THE TRIP CAME AT A PERFECT TIME FOR ME AND I REMEMBER IT WITH PLEASURE.

As I answer my phone one evening, D.O.'s familiar voice: "HI, C'MON OVER." They have returned; D.O. has maintained and enhanced previous progress. All was well as the coffee pot was once again put to constant use. Back to work.

Chapter VI

FORGING AHEAD

More changes. D.O. tried things old, now new. She made chicken salad, assisting with her right hand. All pieces were cut, all ingredients mixed. It took her over an hour to prepare it; it was delicious. "But, Mom," her son said, "you forgot the grapes." I had not anticipated – or known – that in this family, grapes were a key ingredient for chicken salad; with all the work (and pride) she had put into making it, I was shattered by this comment. She was calm.

With all the exercising in Florida – especially the leg movements done in the pool under her husband's direction – the physical therapist declared D.O.'s right leg strong enough to be without the brace! Her first steps – a combination of anxiety and excitement – proved the therapist's evaluation: D.O.'s knee <u>was</u> stable, and she could pull her right foot up enough for her shoe to clear the floor with each step. No more hassles with Velcro straps, broken soles, or squeaky hinges…the brace was stored in the back of her closet!

A new immediate objective was discussed: there was no reason why D.O. could not drive a car again: her reading was sufficient for the written test and her right foot and leg could be controlled well enough. At our urging, D.O. took a driving course and was amazed at the ease of the classroom work (she already knew the material). She had several driving sessions with an instructor.

> TAKING THAT DRIVING COURSE WAS A TOTAL WASTE OF MY TIME AND MONEY. THE INSTRUCTOR ARRIVED WITH A CAR FITTED OUT WITH ALL HAND CONTROLS; WHEN I SAW ALL THE APPARATUS I THOUGHT "THIS IS UNBELIEVABLE FOR ME: I CAN PERFECTLY WELL USE MY RIGHT FOOT ON THE ACCELERATOR" – AND I DID!

She <u>could</u> control her right foot enough to release the accelerator. This had been impossible just a few months before. With repeated exercises she knew how to combat the spasticity and to bring her foot up and out and hold it there – in the case of driving, to release the accelerator.

I took her to the Motor Vehicle Department for the written exam. Forty minutes later she had a 96% correct score. The driving instructor took her for the practical exam; no problem, the license was issued. What a milestone, now on her own!

> IT WAS NO BIG DEAL, GETTING MY LICENSE. I KNEW ALL ALONG THAT I WOULD BE ABLE TO DRIVE. WELL, THAT'S NOT QUITE ACCURATE: I WAS VERY SCARED THE FIRST TIME I DROVE AROUND THE BLOCK WITH MY HUSBAND; I REALLY WASN'T SURE WHETHER I COULD MANAGE IT OR NOT. I WAS SCARED ABOUT

Chapter VI   —   Forging ahead

BEING ABLE TO STEER WITH ONE HAND ON THE WHEEL, AND I DIDN'T KNOW WHETHER I COULD PULL UP FAST ENOUGH WITH MY RIGHT FOOT ON THE ACCELERATOR – OR WHETHER MY RIGHT FOOT WOULD PUSH DOWN ACCIDENTALLY AS IT USED TO WHEN IT WAS SO SPASTIC. AFTER THE FIRST COUPLE OF TIMES DRIVING I KNEW I WOULDN'T HAVE A REAL PROBLEM AND THAT I COULD DO IT SAFELY.

It was fall. It had been almost a year that I had been working with D.O. As the leaves changed, so too did my role. She could manage day-to-day things, and now that she was driving, she needed me less. The physical therapist suggested that I should be with D.O. a few hours every day to assist and encourage exercises and speech and to evaluate problems. And, of course, to bolster morale and note progress. We all agreed.

How can I describe the feeling of tremendous satisfaction we all had as we saw D.O. doing more every day?

She started to take friends out for lunch. She was reading her second novel. Fixing dinner was usually her job once again. And, when I was there, we did exercises old and new, physical and speech. We continued to battle over "to" or "toward," "by" or "in." Sometimes she skipped the most important identifying phrase in telling a story; at my exaggerated look of bewilderment she sighed – and started all over again, sequentially and comprehensively.

The laundry still took an inordinate amount of time. And one time I had the audacity (and insensitivity) to suggest that now that the laundry was completed, we would practice going up and down the stairs. She was horrified and hurt; she <u>had</u> been going up and down; hadn't I noticed? My error. Back off; regroup – and apologize. Grudges and hurts did not last long; among us all was that certain trust which allowed for human foibles. As dusk approached, I was invited for dinner – and quickly accepted.

There were, however, those boundaries of decision-making which were now rightfully hers to decide. D.O.'s anger was real when she learned that I had discussed her cold with the physical therapist and that we, the therapist and I, had cancelled D.O.'s appointment the next day.

> THAT REALLY MADE ME ANGRY. IT REMINDED ME OF THE DOCTOR TALKING TO YOU INSTEAD OF TO ME, ONLY NOW YOU WERE DOING THE SAME THING. AS I RECALL, I TOLD YOU "IF YOU EVER DO THAT AGAIN, YOU'RE FIRED FOR GOOD. THAT WAS MY DECISION TO MAKE, NOT YOURS."

Because I needed full time income, I found three other part-time jobs with those who had suffered a stroke or had other medical problems. My time became structured. D.O., I felt, should be ready to work when I arrived. By the end of November her commitment lagged; it was an almost constant battle of wills to get her to do directed exercises. As my frustration mounted, I decided to take a very calculated risk, to

Chapter VI — Forging ahead

force the issue. I did not consult the family or the specialists: this was between the two of us.

One afternoon, after the second cup of coffee and procrastination, I told D.O. I was quitting. "I am re-hirable, though, whenever you decide to cooperate. I can't be here for a reason each day unless you are ready to work when I arrive; with other jobs, I have to be here and leave at a certain time. Let me know your decision." So hard to say. I left quickly.

Silence. Nothing. I was purposely busy elsewhere the next afternoon when I usually would have been with her. But there were no telephone messages. Had I miscalculated her decision?

The second day it snowed. I stopped at her house on my way between jobs, breezed in, asked her for the shovel. When paths were cleared, she asked what time I would be over tomorrow. "I won't --- You must first agree to continue; it's your decision and commitment I need before I will resume working with you." "O.K., I AGREE." "Fine," I answered, "I'll be here at 1:30 tomorrow afternoon." The crisis had passed; the next day we worked on time.

D.O. saw another specialist doing research on cerebrovascular accidents in terms of blood idiosyncrasies. After extensive tests, a particular medication is advised. Her neurologist disagrees. D.O. was confused and scared about which course to follow. Unfortunately, facing a dilemma like this is not unusual in the medical realm: which physician's advice should be followed in a potentially life-threatening situation. I was upset that anyone should ever find themselves in this situation. Further, D.O., I believed, had enough to cope with on a daily, minute-by-minute basis. After days of questioning, a compromise was reached regarding the suggested medication. Neither physician was entirely content with the compromise, but it was the best solution then, based on the unusual factors of her blood components: the line was fine between hemorrhaging and clotting; she must be monitored constantly. In a real sense she was living with a "loaded gun" at her head.

> THAT WAS A BAD TIME FOR ME. I REALLY DIDN'T KNOW WHOM TO BELIEVE, AND EITHER WAY IT WAS SCARY: IF I DIDN'T TAKE THAT DRUG, I MIGHT GET A BLOOD CLOT AND HAVE ANOTHER STOKE; IF I DID TAKE IT, I MIGHT BLEED TO DEATH. ACTUALLY, I STILL HAVE THE SAME PROBLEM ALTHOUGH I HAVE DIFFERENT MEDICATION TODAY. BUT NO ONE CAN GUARANTEE ANYTHING. WHEN YOU ARE IN THAT REAL SITUATION YOU FEEL ALMOST DESPERATE FOR SOMETHING YOU CAN HOLD ONTO, SOME SENSE OF MEDICAL SECURITY. I GUESS IT'S SOMETHING YOU JUST LEARN HOW TO LIVE WITH.

She talked about her feelings and apprehensions. And with her husband she rejoined a duplicate bridge group as occasional players and usually won.

As lacking as I had been in the beginning of a job description, I was still surprised when different duties seemed to

Chapter VI — Forging ahead

appear – such as catching mice. For some reason there was a rash of them that winter, and D.O. was determined to be rid of them. She didn't know that I had never before set traps and, in fact, really did not like mice at all! It was an exercise in patience (hers) and determined perseverance (mine) as <u>she</u> had to supervise and describe how to set the traps.

> I CAN'T BELIEVE YOU HAD NEVER SET A MOUSETRAP BEFORE! THERE WAS NO WAY I COULD DO IT WITH ONE HAND – AND YOU WITH TWO WEREN'T DOING MUCH BETTER. HOW LONG DID I SPEND, TRYING TO TELL YOU WHAT TO DO? AFTER ABOUT THE TENTH TIME WHEN THE TRAP CAUGHT YOUR FINGERS, YOU MARCHED DOWN TO THE BASEMENT WITH THE FIVE TRAPS AND CHEESE, AND FINALLY CAME UPSTAIRS LOOKING GRIM – BUT, AT LEAST AND AT LAST, EMPTY-HANDED. I HAD TO SMILE: I'D DONE THIS FOR YEARS.

It was not funny an hour later: a trap had sprung. With paper bag in hand I found the caught creature, gingerly grabbed the trap (mouse and all), put it in the bag and took it to her. I refused to do more! With no further ado, D.O. managed to unspring the trap with her left hand, and disposed of its lifeless contents…the first of many such mouse-catching adventures.

Another Christmas was upon us. This year D.O. participated more. And was driving and delivering her presents. And, as she assumed some former roles, there were ongoing family adjustments.

She and I also adjusted – to my daily changing schedule, to her fuller calendar. She went to physical therapy twice a week. She visited friends. She explored weaving. She read voraciously (though her speed was still slower than before her stroke). She did not feel hungry or always remember to eat, even though her sense of taste was back to normal – lettuce and tomatoes and orange juice were now palatable. She would not nap with no reading material beside her; she was stubborn – and gracious – and forging ahead.

Exercises were divided: her list (those she could do without assistance or evaluation) and mine. And whenever she felt particularly put-upon, she went through all those things on her list, and then guessed what was on mine and tried to pre-empt my telling her what to do. My patience ran out as, after an hour one afternoon, I asked if she was finished. "YES, WHEN DO YOU GO TO YOUR NEXT JOB TODAY?" "Not at all," I answered. "OH GOD," she moaned, "I THINK I'LL FIRE YOU AGAIN!" My list was reluctantly attacked.

She had new tools to enable her right hand to hold silverware or a nail file. She showed me how she could (with extreme effort) make small scissors work with the thumb and forefinger of her right hand. It was difficult for me to watch her determination, her grim expression as she willed those fingers into action. The thread was finally cut; she was, deservedly, proud. My eyes were wet with a mixture of sadness at the tremendous effort needed, and joy. I dashed outside to play with the dogs. And the next day I taped a saying cut from a magazine

Chapter VI — Forging ahead

to her mirror: "<u>YOU'VE COME A LONG WAY, BABY --- REPEAT TOMORROW!!</u>" Her eyes were bright with living and daily accomplishments; her friends were more relaxed in her presence. As the days passed, so, too, all the blankets of protection were slowly removed, one by one.

Her eldest daughter moved to California; her youngest daughter was encouraged to move to an apartment. And when her husband was out of town, D.O.'s close friends were aware, but now waited for her to suggest doing things. And each day when I was there for two to three hours I assessed and reacted accordingly. And forever pushed – and swore – and teased – and cajoled – and scolded – and praised – and loved – and pushed, ever onward.

Chapter VII

SETBACKS

It was spring. D.O. and her husband were going to Hawaii for a vacation, and then on to California to visit their eldest daughter. Pleasurable anticipation. No one foresaw the unusual this time. But, it happened, almost, it seemed later, as an unfolding event with succeeding scenes.

> I DIDN'T PARTICULARLY ENJOY HAWAII. ABOUT THE SECOND DAY MY RIGHT LEG BEGAN TO BE NUMB AND PRICKLY, OFF AND ON, AND I REALLY DIDN'T FEEL WELL. THAT EVENING WE WENT TO THE EMERGENCY ROOM AT THE HOSPITAL. AFTER HE EXAMINED ME, THE DOCTOR SAID "I HAVE NEVER SEEN THIS BEFORE: YOU HAVE A UNILATERAL SUNBURN. LOOK, YOUR LEFT SIDE IS FINE, BUT YOUR RIGHT SIDE IS CRIMSON. IF I WERE YOU I WOULD REFRAIN FROM SUNBATHING AS MUCH AS POSSIBLE." NEITHER MY HUSBAND NOR I HAD NOTICED HOW RED MY RIGHT SIDE WAS; THIS HAD NEVER HAPPENED BEFORE, EVEN THE PREVIOUS SUMMER IN FLORIDA WHERE I GOT A GOOD TAN ALL OVER. IN ADDITION TO THE NUMBNESS IN MY LEG AND THE STRANGE SUNBURN, I HAD A BLADDER CONTROL

> PROBLEM. BUT THE DOCTOR COULD OFFER NO FURTHER ADVICE. TEN DAYS LATER WE WENT TO VISIT OUR DAUGHTER IN CALIFORNIA; I STILL DID NOT FEEL WELL.

D.O. had an appointment with a hand specialist to see if there might be anything further that could be done to regain its function. Getting ready at her daughter's on the morning of her scheduled appointment, a grand mal.

> I WASN'T AWARE OF A SEIZURE; I JUST FELT I WAS CRUMBLING. I NEVER IMAGINED I WOULD HAVE A SEIZURE, ESPECIALLY ONE AND A HALF YEARS AFTER MY STROKE. LUCKILY MY DAUGHTER WAS THERE AND FOUND ME ON THE FLOOR.

Convulsions – to the hospital – tests – phone consultations with physician at home – medication – release – home. (There are many forms of epilepsy; its onset is not uncommon after brain injury. The events described here are not necessarily common to all CVA's, however, and are just one person's experience.)

Although I knew, intellectually, that a seizure could occur, and although the physician and physical therapist told me what had happened, still I was unprepared when I saw her: she was in bed, she looked drawn, her speech was poor – halting, searching far more than when she had left for Hawaii. She talked briefly about her grand mal.

Chapter VII — Setbacks

> I DON'T KNOW A THING ABOUT THE ACTUAL SEIZURE. I WOKE UP LYING ON A BED IN THE EMERGENCY ROOM OF A NEARBY HOSPITAL. THERE WAS A VERY NICE LADY DOCTOR WHO TOLD ME THAT I HAD HAD A SEIZURE, AND WE CHATTED UNTIL MY HUSBAND ARRIVED. A STRANGE THING, THOUGH: AFTER THE SEIZURE, THE PROBLEMS WITH MY LEG AND BLADDER COMPLETELY DISAPPEARED.

She was now dizzy <u>all the time</u>, possibly a side effect of the medication I thought. I lied: "You look better than I had expected." I was undone at the toll the seizure seemed to have taken: her muscle power had diminished; she could no longer do a series of motions in exercising her right arm. She was disturbed about this, especially when I broke the series into component parts. I hedged: "it's been a while since you have been doing this exercise. You are also dizzy. Relax!" I did the exercises <u>for</u> her.

> I OFTEN WONDER WHAT THE EFFECTS OF THE FIRST MEDICATION WERE AS COMPARED TO THE EFFECTS OF THE SEIZURE.

She was not allowed to drive anymore. It was too risky in case she had another seizure. Medication would have to control this condition for a long while before she would be able to drive again.

Driving – self-mobility – independence; the hours of concentrated work with her foot and leg and reading which had made it possible. Driving – in one instance, no more.

> I WAS OBVIOUSLY DISAPPOINTED AT NOT BEING ALLOWED TO DRIVE ANYMORE, TO SAY THE LEAST. THE SEIZURE WAS THE LAST STRAW. I DON'T LIKE TO ASK OTHERS TO DRIVE ME: I KNEW WHAT IT WAS TO BE A DRIVER BECAUSE I HAD TAKEN MY MOTHER FOR SPEECH AND PHYSICAL THERAPY AFTER HER FIRST SMALL STROKE A COUPLE OF YEARS AGO. EACH TRIP TOOK ABOUT FOUR HOURS, AND ALTHOUGH I WAS HAPPY TO DO IT, STILL IT WAS A "DRAG." I HATED THE THOUGHT OF HAVING TO ASK PEOPLE TO TAKE ME NOW.

This was my low point. I could make no sense of there being yet another obstacle in her path toward recovery. How much could one person take? For the first time, I had to force myself to go to work, to be with her every day, to do things done long ago in the program. And, once again, I tried to hide my sadness and anger that so much which had been gained with such effort and time should be swept away so quickly.

> AS I SAID BEFORE, THE SEIZURE WAS THE LAST STRAW. AND THEN HAVING MEDICATION NOT RIGHT AND BEING DIZZIER AND DIZZIER EACH DAY WAS UNBEARABLE. EVERY DAY WAS AWFUL FOR THREE WEEKS UNTIL THE MEDICATION WAS CHANGED. THEREAFTER, I WAS NO LONGER DIZZY WHEN I WAS AWAKE, AND I SLEPT TWELVE HOURS A DAY!!

Chapter VII — Setbacks

"No more lying around, we've work to do!" The physical therapist explained about the over-use of weak muscles during the convulsions; how it would take time to build up power again in those muscle groups. It did. Back to exercises of six months ago. "See if you can remember how…" (Sometimes D.O. could, sometimes not). Three friends alternated taking her to therapy three times a week. Speech and motor patterns gradually improved, and D.O. talked quite a bit about the recent past.

> I WON'T FORGET THE REHABILITATION CENTER WHERE I WENT AFTER MY STROKE. IT WASN'T PLEASANT. BUT WHAT COULD I DO ABOUT IT, ESPECIALLY WHEN I COULDN'T MAKE MYSELF UNDERSTOOD?
>
> ONE TIME, ON INSTRUCTIONS OF THE PHYSICAL THERAPIST THERE, I TRIED TO TAKE A FEW STEPS IN MY ROOM BY MYSELF. I FELL, AND COULD NOT GET UP. THE NURSE DISCOVERED ME ON THE FLOOR AND SHE GAVE ME A GOOD TONGUE-LASHING FOR ATTEMPTING TO WALK ALONE. SHE EVEN THREATENED ME WITH BEING TIED IN THE WHEELCHAIR IF I EVER DID IT AGAIN. I COULD NOT TELL HER THAT I WAS ONLY TRYING TO FOLLOW DIRECTIONS.
>
> WHEN YOU CAN'T TALK SUFFICIENTLY, PEOPLE OFTEN TREAT YOU AS INCOMPETENT. THE FIRST FEW DAYS THERE, TWO AIDES WOULD WAKE ME UP AT 5:45 A.M., HELP ME GET DRESSED AND INTO A WHEELCHAIR, AND I WOULD SIT UNTIL

I DID IT! (You did it!!)

BREAKFAST AT 8 A.M. I COULDN'T BELIEVE IT! I DON'T THINK THEY WERE REALLY SUPPOSED TO DO THIS, BUT IT WASN'T UNTIL I GOT SMART AND SAID "NO" FIRMLY ONE MORNING THAT THEY STOPPED GETTING ME UP SO EARLY.

TALKING LOUDLY OR BEING PATRONIZING IS NOT UNUSUAL WHEN PEOPLE DEAL WITH ANYONE WHO SEEMS DIFFERENT. IT DOESN'T JUST HAPPEN TO STROKE PATIENTS; I HAVE SEEN THIS WITH ELDERLY PEOPLE OR THOSE WITH OTHER MEDICAL CONDITIONS SUCH AS PARKINSON'S OR CEREBRAL PALSY FOR EXAMPLE. I DON'T THINK PEOPLE REALIZE HOW MUCH DAMAGE THEY DO TO THE PATIENT. AND, AFTER A WHILE, SOME PATIENTS COME TO EXPECT THIS KIND OF TREATMENT. IT'S HARD TO CORRECT OR CHANGE ATTITUDES – ESPECIALLY WHEN YOU CAN'T COMMUNICATE WELL.

I was upset again, at what I perceived as man's inhumanity to man, unintentional as it may be, especially in a medically-oriented setting. Nothing is perfect – but surely more could be done in staff training to ensure that extra time is taken to try any and all forms of communication when a patient's speech, for example, is drastically impaired, and to respect each person's dignity. I will always wonder whether I would persevere no matter what in a similar situation. "You are exceptional," I tell her; she does not believe this.

DID I EVER TELL YOU ABOUT EATING? EVIDENTLY WHEN THE STROKE PATIENT ENTERS THIS

Chapter VII — Setbacks

REHABILITATION CENTER, TRAYS OF FOOD ARE AUTOMATICALLY SENT UPSTAIRS AND AN AIDE OR TWO IS ASSIGNED TO FEED THE PATIENT. THE FIRST DAY I WAS THERE EVERYBODY WENT DOWNSTAIRS TO THE DINING ROOM – EVERYBODY EXCEPT ME AND ABOUT SIX OTHERS WHO REALLY COULD NOT HANDLE A FORK OR SPOON. I WAS VERY ANGRY BECAUSE I HAD BEEN ABLE TO USE UTENSILS WITH MY LEFT HAND WHILE I WAS IN THE HOSPITAL. BUT, UNTIL I COULD PROVE THAT I WAS CAPABLE OF DOING THIS, I WAS NOT ALLOWED IN THE MAIN DINING ROOM. LOOKING BACK ON IT, IT WAS NO "BIG DEAL;" AT THE TIME, THOUGH, I WAS FURIOUS. AND ON THE SECOND DAY I WENT DOWNSTAIRS WITH EVERYONE ELSE!

WHILE I AM MENTIONING PAST EVENTS I SHOULD TELL YOU, STEVIE, THAT I ALMOST FIRED YOU FOR GOOD LAST SPRING. THAT HAD ALWAYS BEEN MY BUSY TIME, AN OUTDOOR TIME WITH GARDENING, TENNIS, AND BIKING. AND ALL OF A SUDDEN I HAD TO HAVE A HELPER. YOU DON'T KNOW HOW HARD THAT WAS.

I asked her, now, why she hadn't told me this a year ago? "I COULDN'T." (Progress telling me now, at least.)

Over the next two months with continuing work she attained her pre-seizure levels. Her humor and games-playing reappeared and she took advantage of my naiveté. This time I followed her orders to replace any itsy-bitsy ground-cover plants inadvertently removed in weeding her garden (later she laughed as I <u>finally</u> realized her "con" so well executed!) Her color was better, and her eyes bright – and she was restless.

The timing was excellent: her husband had to work in California for a month. It would be a thrilling time, the culmination of a project he had worked on for many years. D.O. would go and be with him.

She was excited, and anxious, remembering the last trip and her seizure there. She did not talk to her husband about her fears and feelings: she did not want to bother him; his work was at a peak. He sensed her reserve, and told me that he felt almost cut off from her, and could not understand why. For several days I thought about this, and decided that they were both protecting each other; that neither D.O. nor her husband was letting on to the other the individual pain each was experiencing in different ways. Feelings seemed to be left unsaid, and sometimes misunderstood.

The day before they left, I lectured them both, together: each had to feel free to talk, to cry; each needed the other. "The protection racket does not work between husband and wife, and it's not fair to either of you. Please don't answer me now; I want you to react with each other." I left with a hasty "Bon Voyage."

D.O. wrote from California. She seemed relaxed. Her husband's work was extremely successful; there were awards and ceremonies in which she participated. She was happy. And, when they returned, there was still more for us to do.

Chapter VIII

NEW TOYS, OLD PROBLEMS, AND INDEPENDENCE

The re-learning process for those who have had a stroke is not short; as soon as one motion or activity is accomplished, there is another – and another – and another to be tried. And tried again. It is a tiring, sometimes boring process in spite of efforts by all to make it otherwise. The temptation for the patient to stop the process is always present; it would be nice to be left alone, to do only those things one felt like doing; to sit back and enjoy rather than face the drudgery of daily progress pressures. D.O. was no exception to these temptations. She <u>was</u> the exception, however, in her usual willingness to keep trying, and in her realization that this was the only way there was if she were to improve. Her husband reinforced this attitude daily. He, too, was exceptional.

D.O. called when she got back from California and said that she wanted to start working again. I saw her the following afternoon and complimented her on initiating the routine; she admitted that she had debated not calling me, but…She talked of the trip, of sharing an apartment with friends; of helping with dinners and dishes. And she still skipped key words ("left-over chicken" in this case) as when telling me, in regard to frugality,

> I HAD TWO BREASTS AND WE PUT THEM IN THE FREEZER.

"You did <u>what</u>?" I asked. She caught her error, laughed, and added:

THEY ARE THAWED OUT NOW!!!

She was not so lively when she saw the latest "toy" I had brought for her to try: a very large rubber ball with a handle, about two and a half feet in diameter. It could be used in many ways: to sit on, to bounce on, to lie on, all of which might help with her trunk balance. She looked askance as I asked her to put her right hand on the handle and try to stand, holding the ball. She could! Next, she tried to pull the ball off the floor, still hanging onto the handle with her right hand. In spite of its size and weight, up it came a good six inches. She was pleased; I was thrilled!

Returning to the pre-trip schedule I arrived mid-afternoon every day and found it hard to catch up, to find out what she had been doing. I needed (and wanted) to know this, especially if she had seen the physical therapist that day (the therapist and I had arranged to alternate areas of exercise between us). And it was necessary to keep probing those areas of thought: current events, attitudes, memory. D.O. all too often turned the discussion so that it was I who was answering her – or being "conned" again.

One midsummer afternoon I asked (told) D.O. to roll her right arm out, something she had been able to do for a long while. "I CAN'T" she said. I was appalled that she used the word "can't." This was not and had not ever been acceptable. But

Chapter VIII — New toys, old problems, and independence

then, I wondered if she had truly forgotten how to initiate this particular motion in her brain? I was ultra-serious as I repeated the directions. She tried it again and again with no result. In desperation, I yelled at her: "Either you are terribly dumb, or (light dawning) you're pulling my leg." She rolled her arm out with ease, gently laughing.

Because she would not give up, those around her were under similar pressure to perform, to read, explore, devise and try anything which might aid in the furtherance of her aims. Thus, the next step became the use of a "biofeedback unit" as a tool toward trying to learn more control of involuntary muscle contractions. Specifically, she would try to learn to consciously decrease the activity of muscles bending her right arm, for example (it was still involuntarily bent most of the time); this would then permit opposing muscles to straighten it. The hope was that once she could relax the spastic muscle groups in her arm and leg she could then keep them relaxed and straight.

By what method a person learns these techniques, even with a unit to measure and show contractions on a dial, is still a mystery to me. I saw her do it with utmost concentration, and marveled. I tried this unit on myself for relaxation and found it near-impossible. It took all of my will power (and a good ten minutes) for me to relax totally. I was exhausted. D.O. watched me and said, "NOW YOU HAVE AN IDEA WHAT I GO THROUGH." Yes.

> I KNEW WHAT I WAS DOING. SOMETIMES IT WORKED, AND SOMETIMES IT DIDN'T, BUT I

KNEW WHY EITHER WAY. WORKING WITH THAT UNIT WAS JUST THAT, WORK. I WAS QUITE DRAINED AFTER EACH SESSION. BUT I KNEW THAT IF I COULD LEARN TO RELAX CERTAIN MUSCLES I WOULD BE ABLE TO CONTROL MY ARM AND LEG BETTER.

After several sessions at the therapist's she rented a biofeedback unit for home use. Although not always successful, she did learn over the next few months the technique of muscle-relaxation. It showed in her gait and her right arm which was now straighter on most occasions. The ability (and mental effort) to walk normally took on greater meaning as I began to realize all the components she has to keep in mind, sequentially, with each step. Walking, probably the most complex motor activity we do (and take for granted).

We all knew that none of this was fun: it was constant effort and experimentation. We walked outside with me facing her, holding hands to try to get the walking rhythm and balance. Concentration was the key, and the habit of concentration each time D.O. walked was hard to instill. We tried walking barefoot on a beach; the sand was hot and walking uphill <u>was</u> a challenge! Or we walked around the block and she had to describe what she saw along the way at the same time – split concentration, very difficult for D.O. to accomplish. But she tried, and kept trying.

Just as she was absorbing and using new techniques, so, too, she was doing more. She and her husband rejoined the duplicate

Chapter VIII — *New toys, old problems, and independence*

bridge group on a regular basis once a month. All of a sudden she was to have this group – sixteen – for dinner, and insisted that she would do all the preparation by herself. (The dinner was a huge success; she and her husband won at bridge.) She was reading books regularly. And she could now describe their content and her reactions, or argue thoughtfully if she disagreed with an author's premise.

> IF I HAVE TIME I READ A LOT. IF I READ A NOVEL STRAIGHT THROUGH IT TAKES THREE TO FOUR DAYS, DEPENDING, OF COURSE, ON WHAT IT IS.

When I arrived each day I usually knew within five minutes when something was bothering her: not only was her conversation more stilted, but spasticity still showed in her right leg and arm. By fall she could usually identify problems when I asked why she was upset.

> IT'S CALLED APPREHENSION. TODAY, FOR INSTANCE, FIRST I WENT TO THE HAIRDRESSER. THEN TONIGHT WE ARE GOING TO THE SYMPHONY FOR THE FIRST TIME SINCE MY STROKE. I CAN'T REMEMBER HOW THE STAIRS ARE OR EXACTLY WHERE OUR SEATS ARE.

I reminded her that until now she could not pinpoint her worries, and the fact she could now identify them was another huge accomplishment. I suggested that she pat herself on the back (with her right hand, of course!) a thousand times every night: she had learned more than some people ever learn. I told her she was impressive; she was dubious.

For D.O., frustrations we all face in daily living were far more aggravating, and people were not always considerate. She had to call a local business about her son's account:

> A WOMAN ANSWERED IN A VERY BUSINESS-LIKE MANNER, AND I STARTED TO DESCRIBE THE PROBLEM. I GUESS I WAS RATTLED AND DIDN'T TALK FAST ENOUGH: SHE HUNG UP ON ME. I WAS REALLY UPSET. I WENT INTO THE LIVING ROOM AND TRIED TO THINK WHAT I SHOULD DO; MY HUSBAND WAS OUT OF TOWN, MY SON WAS AWAY AT COLLEGE, AND I KNEW IT WOULD TAKE WEEKS FOR MY SON TO STRAIGHTEN IT OUT BY LETTER. SO, I PLANNED EXACTLY WHAT I WOULD SAY AND MEMORIZED IT IN MY HEAD. I CALLED AGAIN. THIS TIME I PLUNGED RIGHT IN, REMEMBERING WHAT I WANTED TO SAY AND THE WOMAN FINALLY UNDERSTOOD ME.

I usually stopped between other jobs to check and see if there were errands I could do on my way. Sometimes we went out for lunch, depending on our schedules, but always I was with D.O. mid-afternoon, the constant reminder of specifics to be done. Occasionally I would arrive to find the door locked and a note indicating she had gone out with friends. Another adjustment – and worry lest she overdid and became overtired. I told her how pleased I was whenever she was busy, but that she did not always need to push herself to the point of discomfort or

Chapter VIII — *New toys, old problems, and independence*

exhaustion. Organizing her schedule so that there was always a good rest period was not one of her priorities, this was "not normal," and she resented my insinuations when she had been out and about all day.

> IF I AM NOT BUSY, I WILL TRY TO HAVE A QUIET PERIOD DURING THE DAY. BUT IF I AM BUSY, THEN TO HECK WITH IT: I WOULD RATHER BE DOING THINGS. AND IF I GET OVERTIRED, WELL, THEN I WILL REST LATER. BY THE WAY: I GENERALLY DO LIE DOWN FOR HALF AN HOUR EACH DAY.

She began entertaining occasionally and accompanying her husband on short business trips around the country. On one such jaunt, this time to Hampton, Virginia, they attended a banquet with several hundred people. As she retold it later with great pleasure:

> THE DINNER WAS IN THE LARGE BANQUET HALL. I WALKED ALL THE WAY DOWN TO THE OTHER END TO GET MY DINNER, AND CARRIED IT ALL THE WAY BACK, WITHOUT MY CANE. I WAS PERFECTLY RELAXED!

Such pride well deserved. "Coffee, Madam?" "YES."

We had lots of coffee. Each of us knew another chapter must soon be closed; it was time for me to move on. We talked of things past – of the funnies and not-so-funnies; of the tremendous progress she had made. Again, I told her that she was exceptional; she still did not believe it.

She knew that the physical therapist was cutting her sessions to once a week (would she be able to maintain her progress essentially by herself?) She did not yet know that the physician, therapist and I have discussed and calculated the necessary risk of eliminating D.O.'s outside support systems; she had to stand alone – and decide for herself what kind of help she <u>really</u> needed.

There were days when her gait was bad (but she could still walk), or when her speech was less comprehensible (but she could still talk). She continued to have trouble processing more than one conversation at a time, or following if someone spoke too fast. She recognized this, and could now interrupt with a "say it again, please" to indicate her confusion. She forgot telephone messages and caused unrest – and apologized. She was addressing and sending a few Christmas cards this year.

And, oh, the shopping (as if to make up for the past two Christmases). Such pleasure for her – and for all of us, watching.

About ten days before Christmas her husband asked her if she would like her present early? "I talked to the doctor today. He says you can drive again – <u>now</u>." Tears of joy as independent mobility reappeared and her world re-opened. And another example of her husband's initiative at the perfect time.

> OF COURSE I WAS THRILLED TO BE ABLE TO DRIVE AGAIN. IT HAD BEEN VERY FRUSTRATING NOT TO BE ABLE TO GET OUT WHENEVER I

Chapter VIII — New toys, old problems, and independence

> WANTED, AND IT HAD BEEN WORSE AFTER THE SEIZURE WHEN I HAD HAD TO GIVE IT UP.

I braced myself for what soon must be: the goal of long ago when I would work myself out of a job and would have done what I had tried to do – aid in the process of regaining independence of living.

> THE CHILDREN WERE ALL HOME FOR THE HOLIDAYS. WITH ALL THE ACTIVITY (AND DRIVING!) I DECIDED NOT TO HAVE YOU OVER THAT WEEK; I HAD OTHER THINGS I WANTED TO DO!!

New Year's Eve Day, 1976: I was invited over for coffee. We exchanged chat about our respective Christmases. There was a pause. I did not anticipate the role-reversal; <u>D.O. was counseling me</u> about finding another job. It was all I could do to remain calm; I told her that one way or another I would be employed elsewhere within a month.

D.O. called several days later wondering where I was, and during that month I was still with her part-time. We patted each other on the back and supported our separate endeavors. I watched her continue to use the biofeedback unit, and occasionally helped her set it up. Her directions for the placement of the electrodes were precise; her knowledge of what nerve triggered what muscle contraction and limb motion which would result was impressive. I told her this; she shrugged as if to discount the hours and hours spent working.

WHENEVER I AM LOW I TRY TO THINK OF ALL THOSE WHO ARE WORSE OFF THAN I. AT LEAST I AM PROGRESSING, AND THIS IS AN ADDED IMPETUS TO KEEP GOING, TO KEEP TRYING. NO ONE KNOWS ALL THE ANSWERS, BUT I FEEL SORRY FOR SOME STROKE PATIENTS WHO HAVE GIVEN UP, WHO ARE NOT FORCED – YES, FORCED – TO TRY TO DO, TO TRY TO SPEAK, TO TRY TO THINK. I WONDER IF THEY KNOW WHAT A BURDEN THEY ARE TO OTHERS AND WHETHER, IF THEY KNEW, THEY MIGHT BE SHAMED INTO ACTIVITY AND EFFORT. I KNEW WHAT A BURDEN I WAS AT FIRST, AND I SAID TO MYSELF "I'LL BE DAMNED IF I'LL STAY LIKE THIS FOREVER!" BUT I WAS LUCKY: MY FAMILY, THE SPECIALISTS AND YOU ALL AGREED AND MADE ME WORK AT <u>EVERYTHING</u>, AND FOR THAT I AM GRATEFUL.

I smiled, thinking back, remembering how difficult it was to be the enforcer, how wrenching the effort and frustration. But, what satisfactions for all to see and hear the consequences of those forced efforts.

All was not work that month: We spent a day shopping with a long, relaxed lunch in the middle. Invariably whenever we were out in public and momentarily separated, someone asked me, "Who is that lovely young woman? She has such sparkle." They did not always realize that she had had a stroke. It happened over and over. And when I told these compliments to

Chapter VIII — New toys, old problems, and independence

D.O., she blushed; I hope she felt the pride of accomplishment. This happened again today as we proceeded from one end of the enclosed shopping center to the other, stopping, picking out, and trying on. Sales personnel were uniformly gracious and helpful. And, all the while, we talked.

"Over a year ago when I 'quit' you should know that that was a very scary time for <u>me</u>, waiting to hear from you. I had to force you to reassess and to recommit yourself to working a few hours a day. But, no way was I <u>really</u> quitting then; you were not ready for that."

"AND, TODAY?" D.O. asked.

"Today, lady, no problem: I am certain you can cope!"

Chapter IX

NOTES FROM JOURNAL, FEBRUARY 1977

In the beginning I saw this job as a challenge to help someone regain as much function and speech capability as possible. Today I can honestly say that I've had a role. The rewards have been tremendous. I will always be grateful for the team situation with the specialists; with no prior specific medical training or CVA experience I had much to learn.

I know that the idea of seeing me less produces a tinge of unease for my friend. But, like a graduation, the idea of my moving on is also anticipated pleasure. And relief from having an extra person around the house; once more home will be D.O.'s own domain in which to do or not do as *she* desires. There is no question in my mind that she will prosper, given the chance and the confidence of those around her.

We "held hands" these past two and a half years, she and I. I dare say she has led me just as much as I her, if not more so. The books will never be balanced even-steven (but then they seldom are.)

There are still problems. There may always be problems to greater or lesser extents. The blood-clotting factor will always have to be watched. Her fatigue level is still apparent and she still should learn to readily and automatically deal with this (*my* biggest concern). She will probably always have residual speech and spasticity problems when tired or uneasy. And I hope that she develops some interests where her boundless intellect, creativity and warmth have a chance to give strength and confidence to others in a satisfying way for her.

The family support was and is exceptional. There will always be periods, moments, of remembrances past, of how things used to be and no longer are. But the basics of love are there and stronger, the family unit is more cohesive despite distances of children's abodes.

As I write her a note of thanks, I end with a quote from a song I wrote for her:

"Please keep the coffee warming,

'Cause I'll be 'round, no warning, to say

'Hi, friend, and how are you?' and

'My, friend, what you can do <u>new</u>!!'"

Chapter X

EIGHT MONTHS LATER

She <u>is</u> coping! And she is reshaping her life. Little things are not as important as they once were; her philosophy has changed: life is short and unpredictable; "I'll try it, now." She is still pushing onward and is not always gentle on herself; I give her hell.

She has taken several long trips, some successful and others not so. This spring she rejoined her ceramic group. As this had been her real creative love years ago, I was apprehensive lest she find the frustration of working with one hand unbearable. I should not have worried; although her large dish took twice the amount of time to fashion, and although she was exhausted by the effort, she was artistically pleased with the outcome of her original design and the experience was satisfying. She continues with the class once a week.

After weeks of self-doubt she started horseback riding. It had been discussed as a possibility months before, and was now urged by the physical therapist, principally as a benefit to the muscles of her right leg. On the side was the hope for enjoyment of a sport in which she had participated many years ago. And, it could be another social outlet. Collective breaths are held – needlessly.

THE FIRST COUPLE OF TIMES I TOOK LESSONS I WAS IN A RING WITH THE INSTRUCTOR. BUT AFTER THE FIRST HALF HOUR I WAS POSTING IN THE ENGLISH SADDLE, <u>WITHOUT HANGING ON</u>! WE WENT ON TRAILS THE NEXT TIME; HE SHOWED ME HOW I COULD GO DOWN A STEEP BANK AND THROUGH THE CANAL AND UP THE OTHER SIDE WITH NO PROBLEM. ALTHOUGH I RODE WITH AN ENGLISH SADDLE AND LEARNED TO POST, I USUALLY HAD BOTH REINS IN MY LEFT HAND AND "NECK-REINED" THE HORSE. I USED THE SAME HORSE EACH TIME: HE WAS VERY PATIENT AND WELL-TRAINED. THE ONLY THING I COULD NOT DO NORMALLY WAS TO GET ON – OR OFF – THE HORSE: THERE WAS NO WAY THAT I COULD KEEP MY BALANCE WHILE PUTTING MY LEFT FOOT UP INTO THE STIRRUP; NOR COULD I THROW MY RIGHT LEG OVER THE HORSE FROM THAT ANGLE. WE DEVISED A SYSTEM USING A BALE OF STRAW: ONCE I GOT UP ON THAT AND WAS HIGHER, I COULD MOUNT UP WITHOUT TOO MUCH DIFFICULTY.

Ignoring her protests, I insisted that she have a good helmet for riding. She went to a local shop, and came back with one that was inferior: it had no chin strap. Fearful that if she fell she might really injure her head, I called all over town until a professional model was located. With English boots, britches and helmet, she looked the experienced horsewoman; I soon discovered that she really could ride.

Chapter X — Eight months later

The first time I went riding with her I was less than calm: the instructor was ill and could not accompany us. D.O. decided we would go anyway! My horse's stride was longer than hers, and after about fifteen minutes I looked back over my shoulder to see her heading back toward the barn. Thoughts raced through my head: was she all right? Why had she turned around? Or had her horse decided to go home and she could not control him? By the time I caught up with her she had turned onto another trail. "What's the matter?" "YOU MISSED THE TRAIL!" she answered matter-of-factly.

That summer I rode with her once a week. One time her son and a friend came, too. I saw her stay on when inadvertently galloping. And sometimes I looked at the right moment and saw her holding her reins in her right (affected) hand while swatting a fly with her left – or her right arm, relaxed, and resting on her thigh. <u>Fantastic</u>!

She went to an out-of-town specialist to see if she could be a candidate for an experimental "gadget." It would trigger an electrical impulse to help her stabilize her right ankle. Nothing like this was available locally although some hospitals in the East, we later discovered, use this unit automatically after a trauma affecting mobility. She was declared eligible, and looks forward to its arrival in a few months.

Her schedule is full. Houseguests keep appearing and staying. She has revived picnic suppers on the beach. All who see her marvel at the long way she has come, at her vivaciousness and interest in all that goes on around her, at her courage. She goes out for dinner, entertains her husband's business associates and wives; she goes to the theater or the symphony or to watch pro tennis.

> EVERY DAY I FIND OUT SOMETHING NEW. MANY IS THE DAY I WAKE UP AND THINK "I'M ALIVE! IT'S ANOTHER DAY!!"

I see her often. For my part, the temptation to suggest she try something a different way is always present; old habits are hard to lose and I do battle with myself to hold my tongue (not always successful). Similarly, I miss the daily exercises, the chance to watch as minute muscles flicker. I suspect she knows my inner battles.

The unusual still occurs. Her blood specialist died suddenly, and D.O. is faced, on the one hand with sadness, and on the other with that very real fear: who is able to carry on the research? Specifically, to whom can she turn with her special clotting problem? On the advice of friends she makes an appointment with another physician who was the specialist's associate. Her patient records are transferred prior to her visit, and he has been told about her. Once again, fallibility is demonstrated:

> I WALKED INTO HIS OFFICE AND CASUALLY PLACED MY CANE IN MY RIGHT HAND (Note: she holds it in the hand so badly affected, a great achievement). HE GREETED ME, AND ASKED "HOW ARE YOU DOING WITH YOUR LEFT ARM

Chapter X — Eight months later

AND HAND?" IT WAS OBVIOUS THAT HE HAD NOT READ MY RECORDS. I DID NOT CORRECT HIM, MENTALLY DISMISSING HIS FURTHER REMARKS ON MY HEALTH. I NEVER RETURNED.

I am appalled at her description of this consultation, and tell her that I feel like storming into that office with righteous accusations. D.O., however, tells me that I am over-reacting (again), that it is <u>her</u> problem, and that anger will not lead to a solution.

I SAW THE WRONG PERSON, PERIOD. SOMEWHERE ALONG THE LINE THERE WILL BE A BETTER ANSWER TO MY PROBLEM. IN THE MEANTIME, I HAVE OTHER THINGS TO DO. AND I WILL KEEP MY EARS OPEN!

Chapter XI

EPILOGUE

It is four and a half years since D.O. suffered her stroke. She continues to improve. Her progress is less dramatic now, but progress there is. She attended a cooking class and is relying less on frozen foods; as before her stroke, she is creating interesting meals and is often asked for her recipes. Once a week she goes to ceramic class; she is able to throw five pounds of clay on the wheel with her left hand. She has made pots, and several plates to match a set she made years ago. People are urging her to consider selling these one-of-a-kind items.

There are many things she still wants to be able to do. Uppermost are riding a bicycle, eating with her right hand, and walking better. And yet the tediousness of exercise is sometimes its own obstacle; resolves to work each day are not always carried out.

> BUT IT DOESN'T MAKE SENSE: I KNOW WHAT I HAVE TO DO, AND I WANT TO DO IT, BUT I DON'T DO IT AS OFTEN AS I SHOULD AND I DON'T KNOW WHY. BUT IF I DON'T GET BETTER I WILL BE DEVASTATED.

The dichotomy of "if I work I can improve" versus "I'm tired of working" produces discontent and anxiety; in this D.O. is normal: we all wrestle with these opposites in our own lives. Usually, though, we rationalize away our "shoulds" versus "wants." D.O., however, can't ignore them now: they are magnified, and part of her everyday life.

So, too, are the struggles she still has with those daily routines most people take for granted. Changing the bed, taking out the trash – those household chores of laundry or shopping, and carrying the grocery sacks with one hand – all these take considerable thought and effort and time, even now. Often I find myself forgetting this fact of her life, only to be quickly reminded as she describes a day's events. I wonder how many people realize the time and energy it takes for D.O. to complete these routine things? She seldom complains; things which don't work out the way she had anticipated are told offhandedly. And, even after a "disastrous" day, she manages, somehow, to regroup, and to try the same things the next day. And the next.

Today D.O. is functioning within her limitations and still working to lessen them. Her husband says that she is a better communicator than she was before her stroke, that her slower speech is a mixed blessing: it makes others really listen to what she is saying; and because she has to think out what she wants to say, she speaks more precisely than all of us.

She lives for today and is eager to try anything, today. And, like others who have survived a traumatic medical experience, she has learned to live with the fear of dying which is always present. It is a different kind of fear than most of us know; it is specific.

Chapter XI — Epilogue

> I DON'T FEAR DEATH SO MUCH AS I DON'T WANT TO DIE. I USUALLY DON'T THINK ABOUT IT. BUT, WHENEVER ANYTHING STRANGE HAPPENS – A DIFFERENT PAIN, OR THE SEIZURE A FEW YEARS AGO, OR IF MY LEG OR ARM GO TO SLEEP – MY FIRST THOUGHT IS "OH MY GOD, IS THIS IT, AM I ABOUT TO HAVE ANOTHER STROKE AND DIE?" I CAN'T EXPLAIN IT BETTER EXCEPT TO SAY THAT IT IS MUCH MORE REAL AND IMMEDIATE WHEN YOU KNOW THAT IT REALLY COULD HAPPEN.

I know my panic whenever something untoward happens to her, and I wonder how she and so many others manage to submerge this fear on a day-to-day basis. The importance of others' care and support can not be emphasized enough. Those with similar problems speak of little things and how grateful they are for a phone call, an unplanned visit, a simple "Hi, how are you?" These are no longer little things; they tell me their meaning is magnified. And appreciated.

The adjustment from an active, community-involved, independent pattern to a more arduous and less mentally stimulating one takes time. Satisfactions of newly-learned tasks do not always compensate for the loss of former activities. D.O. identifies these frustrations, and is searching for further meaningful activity which will be intellectually challenging yet within her lowered endurance level. In the meantime she is cataloging a small library of medical and sociological texts on a volunteer basis. Sometimes she helps with large mailings:

folding, stuffing, licking envelopes. But her special talent is helping others find solutions to procedural problems, or those involving interpersonal relations. Her perspective is focused, and she seems to have a sixth sense, an uncanny knack for pinpointing real issues. I take advantage of this skill often.

She is initiating contact with people who have, for whatever reason, drifted. It is hard.

> TODAY I AM APPALLED AT MY LACK OF UNDERSTANDING OF MY MOTHER'S PROBLEMS AFTER HER FIRST STROKE. AND, JUST AS SHE WAS AWARE OF OTHER PEOPLE'S NON-UNDERSTANDING, SO TOO, I CAN SPOT THOSE PEOPLE WHO STILL DO NOT ACCEPT MY STROKE.

Relationships with past friends are sometimes not smooth, and she worries about this. She is sensitive and wonders why when some decline repeated invitations. I point out the natural inclination to protect her, to avoid subjects in which her participation is now only vicarious; or the tendency of others to skip telling her <u>their</u> problems which, in comparison to what she has been through, seem trivial. We talk of the difficulty others have because they are not comfortable. She is not sure what she can do to enhance these friendships; there is no easy answer. Repeatedly she is assured by family and close friends that she is loved (not just tolerated), and that she still has the same qualities people saw in her before her stroke: compassion, intelligence, and that certain "joie de vivre." She thinks about this, and sorts her own feelings and alternatives.

Chapter XI — Epilogue

Her venturesome spirit is unquenchable. Recently she went with three others to sample a physical isolation tank – the current leisure-time activity with an hour of floating and relaxation in an individual tank of salt water. Each tank was separated and covered, each person in their own dark and liquid world. D.O. had the best time of all; for while the others worried about her safety, whether she could get out of the tank by herself, she spent the hour floating in relative comfort. When told later of the others' concern, she was genuinely surprised – and secretly pleased.

She is sometimes stubborn to the point of exasperation. She will not always say when she is tired, or ask for help; "I can manage" is her standard retort. Repeatedly I suggest that whenever others are around, she should let them help: they need to feel needed, I remind her. Further, she should save her own energy for more important things than routine household necessities. These suggestions are not often acted upon. Occasionally I scream!

A left-footed accelerator was installed in her car, a safety measure for long driving hours or for when D.O. is tired. But she still shifts gears, with her left hand: that is one control she refuses to have changed. "I can manage shifting perfectly," she says archly. "I don't <u>need</u> a left-handed gear control!"

D.O. complains whenever anyone does anything which could be interpreted as solicitous of her slower mobility or maneuverability. Whenever I pull my feet in as she is going by my chair, she objects. I tell her I am just being polite, that I do the same for anyone. "You're oversensitive. Knock it off!" I say, mimicking her.

There is a fine line between being friendly, concerned, and over-protective. It is difficult to remind her to eat, for example; she seems to have lost her sense of hunger and often forgets this necessity. There are only so many ways one can ask her if she has had lunch – a monotonous question, a protective concern. One day I plunged right in when she answered the telephone: "I am your stomach. Have you fed me today?" – the one and only time the question has been received with laughter rather than put-upon indignation.

Since working with D.O. I have been acquainted with about twenty other stroke patients, some on a working level. I have observed varying degrees of success in terms of the regaining of function and independence. There seem to be several keys to the degree one adjusts and determines to exert the necessary daily effort toward the goal of independence. Critical, of course, is the precise location of brain damage. But, given a still rational mind with fairly logical thought processes, and some minimal use of muscles, the presence – or lack of – individual motivation carries one through, or doesn't.

In D.O.'s case, she was able early on, with her husband's assistance, to accept the fact that for any progress she would have to work and work <u>hard</u>, everyday. Her basic intelligence and sense of humor were (and are) invaluable, not just pleasant

Chapter XI — Epilogue

attributes. Above all, the never-give-up support and love of her family were and are steadfast and verbal. They continue to goad and push her toward more recovery and function; they are united in not accepting the status quo. They <u>know</u> she <u>can</u> do better.

> WHAT ALTERNATIVE DID I HAVE? A NURSING HOME? NO WAY! I HAD TO WORK, PERIOD. MY HUSBAND SAID "GET WITH IT!" I DID, NOT ALWAYS EAGERLY.
>
> AND BY THE WAY: SELDOM DID MY FAMILY – OR YOU FOR THAT MATTER – FINISH SENTENCES FOR ME: YOU ALL WAITED. I <u>HAD</u> TO TRY OR IT WOULD HAVE BEEN AWFULLY QUIET! THE SAME HELD TRUE FOR DOING THINGS: SOMETIMES YOU SHOWED ME HOW, SOMETIMES I FIGURED IT OUT, BUT YOU MADE ME TRY TO DO WHATEVER IT WAS BY MYSELF. IT DIDN'T MATTER HOW IT WAS DONE AS LONG AS I DID IT. I HATED BEING PUSHED TO DO THINGS, BUT I CERTAINLY LEARNED A LOT IN A HURRY BECAUSE I HAD NO OTHER CHOICE: NO ONE ELSE WOULD DO THEM.
>
> YOU KNOW, EACH STROKE PATIENT IS DIFFERENT: SOME PEOPLE HAVE SMALL STROKES, SOME HAVE BIG; SOME AT 20 YEARS OLD, OTHERS AT 60. NINE TIMES OUT OF TEN PEOPLE AREN'T REALLY CONSCIOUSLY AWARE THAT SOMETHING DISABLING LIKE A STROKE COULD AFFECT THEM – UNTIL IT HAPPENS. AND,

IF I COULD GIVE ADVICE TO THOSE WHO HAVE SUFFERED A STROKE IT WOULD BE "<u>YOU'VE GOT TO FIGHT, JUST FIGHT, AND KEEP ON FIGHTING</u>. AND WHILE YOU ARE TRYING TO LEARN HOW TO DO THINGS DIFFERENTLY, DON'T SAY TO YOURSELF 'IT IS IMPOSSIBLE', OR 'I CAN'T': IF ANYONE TELLS YOU THIS, SCRATCH THAT PERSON OFF YOUR LIST AND LISTEN TO SOMEONE ELSE. DON'T EVER LET ANYONE TELL YOU THAT X, Y, Z IS THE MOST YOU WILL BE ABLE TO DO.

AND JUST AS YOU MUST TRY DOING THINGS, YOU MUST TRY SPEAKING, TOO. DO NOT LET OTHERS SPEAK FOR YOU: IT IS AN EASY HABIT TO FALL INTO. BUT THIS WILL ONLY PROLONG THE TIME IT WILL TAKE TO LEARN HOW TO TALK AGAIN. SURE, YOU WILL MAKE MISTAKES – I DID AND STILL DO – BUT IT'S THE ONLY WAY. AND WHEN WORDS COME OUT WRONG, SMILE TO YOURSELF AND START ALL OVER AGAIN."

WHILE THIS BOOK WAS TAKING SHAPE I DID A GREAT DEAL OF THINKING ABOUT THOSE AREAS I BELIEVE ARE CRITICAL IN A STROKE PATIENT'S REHABILITATION. IT GOES WITHOUT SAYING THAT THE LOVE AND SUPPORT OF THOSE CLOSEST TO YOU ARE INDISPENSABLE. IN MY CASE, IT WAS RARE WHEN MY HUSBAND OR THOSE AROUND ME LET ME GET AWAY WITH AN

Chapter XI — Epilogue

UNFINISHED SENTENCE OR A NEGATIVE PHRASE. THE ATTITUDES OF FAMILY AND SPECIALISTS MAKE ALL THE DIFFERENCE AS YOU BEGIN TO LEARN ALL OVER AGAIN HOW TO TAKE CARE OF YOURSELF, HOW TO TALK, HOW TO LIVE WITH WHATEVER DISABILITIES YOU NOW HAVE.

<u>THE PEOPLE AROUND A STROKE PATIENT SHOULD KEEP AN OPEN MIND</u>. FOR EXAMPLE, IF THE PATIENT SAYS "LET'S TRY X, Y, OR Z," I WOULD ADVISE THOSE PEOPLE TO GO ALONG WITH IT – IT MIGHT WORK! OFTEN THE PATIENT KNOWS BEFORE ANYONE ELSE WHAT NEXT STEP IS POSSIBLE. I HAVE HEARD OF FAMILIES AND SPECIALISTS WHO ASSUME THAT A STROKE PATIENT WILL NEVER BE ABLE TO DO CERTAIN THINGS; THIS ATTITUDE, I BELIEVE, IS DETRIMENTAL: EVERY CVA IS DIFFERENT, AND NO WAY CAN YOU PREDICT WHAT WILL BE POSSIBLE – <u>NOBODY KNOWS UNLESS YOU TRY IT OUT</u>. IT IS EASY TO SPOT THOSE PEOPLE WHO MAKE THESE ASSUMPTIONS, AND I WISH I COULD TELL THEM HOW SHATTERING THEY ARE TO THE PATIENT. <u>DON'T PRESUME A THING</u> – I CAN'T EMPHASIZE THIS ENOUGH. IT APPLIES TO ALL DOCTORS AND THERAPISTS, AND TO ANYONE WHO IS WORKING IN A PROFESSIONAL SETTING. OBVIOUSLY, THIS SAME ADVICE HOLDS TRUE FOR THE FAMILY OF A STROKE VICTIM – AND EVEN FOR A FRIEND. <u>MOST IMPORTANT OF</u>

<u>ALL, RULE NUMBER ONE IS: TREAT US, LIKE ANYONE, AS HUMAN BEINGS, PERIOD.</u>

There is another dimension which needs inclusion: her husband and three grown children could not have been more supportive as I tried in any way possible to push, urge, and goad their wife and mother. When a virtual stranger all of a sudden becomes an eight-hour-a-day fixture, the temptation is for a family to protect the patient-member, to tell the "stranger" in subtle and not-so-subtle ways that we, the family, know much more than you could ever know about this person. The implication here is that although it may be nice to have the stranger helping, still, there are boundaries to responsibilities and concerns – specific areas are "off limits" to all but the family. I have experienced this attitude in other work circumstances and am convinced that these protective walls create a real barrier to the rehabilitation process and to the dedication of anyone trying to help. <u>This never happened here.</u> Moreover, I was not told until recently of the many evenings when D.O. vented much anger about me – such as "She's pushing me too hard," or "She doesn't understand." or "She's not fair." Once again, the family was unusual: they did not budge in their support on my behalf.

> STEVIE, YOU WERE THERE, PERIOD – EVEN WHEN I SAW MY DOCTOR! I OFTEN TRIED TO GET RID OF YOU, BUT I DIDN'T HAVE A THING TO SAY ABOUT IT…(WELL ALMOST!)

Chapter XI — Epilogue

In retrospect, I am grateful for this unity and support without which my effectiveness would have been greatly reduced and, I suspect, my friend's recovery process slower.

The professional "team" still exists in that each member still cares and is aware of how things are going. D.O. sees the physical therapist fairly regularly, and, of course, the neurologist – less frequently but regularly; and, occasionally, the speech therapist. Periodically I run into one or the other and we exchange marvels at the strides she still makes. It was (and is) a real team, not just names on paper; <u>no one (family included) cared who did what as long as all conferred and as long as the patient's progress was enhanced and continuing</u>. Professional jealousies were non-existent; each was free to consult the others at any time. Needless to say, I consulted – often.

My on-the-job training was immediate, and has carried over to similar care-giving employment. I learned to be more aware, to observe constantly. Without my seeing, sensing, hearing, there could have been accidents; without some sense of D.O.'s mood it would have been difficult (if not impossible) to judge, to evaluate, to mesh and to goad. I needed to be involved in order to empathize, and to try to make sense out of some things nonsensical. That I cared as a casual friend to start with kept me on the job during those first few days of personal horror at the effects of the stroke, coupled with an acute sense of inexperience in that field. That D.O. and I became close friends is a matter of chance and choice. I sensed early on that D.O. and I could easily become "enemies": you know someone awfully well when you are together 8-10 hours a day, five days a week. I was careful; so was she – and we used to joke that all this time together was "worse than being married."

> SERIOUSLY, THOUGH, I HOPE THAT WHAT WE HAVE SAID IN THESE PAGES WILL GIVE OTHERS THINGS TO THINK ABOUT AND WORK FOR. IT'S A LONG, SOMETIMES PAINFUL HAUL, FOR THE PATIENT AND FOR EVERYONE CONCERNED. IT IS WORK, ALWAYS. FOR ALL THOSE SIMILARLY AFFLICTED, LET ME URGE THEM TO KEEP AT IT!

Each day brings its triumphs. D.O. mentions that "YESTERDAY I DROVE TO..." (A city fifty miles distant). "By yourself?" I ask. "OF COURSE," she answers. I make her stop her narrative and heap praise: who would have thought a few short years ago that she would be taking off like this on her own? Her reaction is immediate: "WELL, <u>WHY NOT</u>?!!"

The weeks go on. The world goes on. So does she.

She is unusual, this woman I know. For, as she said with emphasis one night as we discussed again her continuing progress,

> I'M NOT A QUITTER!

ADDENDUM

It is always risky to write about medical conditions and happenings. This book is not meant to be a "How To" book in specific techniques for anyone having a speech or physical difficulty. We urge those having problems, or those who think they may be having problems, to contact specialists who have been trained to diagnose and prescribe appropriate treatment modalities.

I DID IT! (You did it!!)

BOOK ORDERS

To order copies of "I DID IT! (You did it!!)" complete the form below and mail it with your check to:

>   Ms. S. Lesher
>   5780 South Cherokee Street
>   Littleton, CO 80120-2339

Within Colorado		**Outside Colorado**	
Price	$16.00	Price	$16.00
Colorado Sales Taxes	$1.60	No Sales Taxes	
Shipping and Handling	$2.10	Shipping and Handling	$2.10
TOTAL per book	$19.70	TOTAL per book	$18.10
Number of copies	_____	Number of copies	_____
Total Amount remitted	_____	Total Amount remitted	_____

Please allow two weeks for delivery.

Name_____

Address_____

City_____State_____Zip_____

AUTHORS

Stevia W. Sargent Lesher ("Stevie") is a graduate of the Shipley School and of Mt. Holyoke College, 1955, with a major in economics and sociology. After marrying, she was a bookmobile librarian in rural eastern Kentucky, and moved to the Denver area in 1959. She served as an officer on the Boards of the YWCA of Metropolitan Denver, Elementary School PTO, a school district Parents' Council, and County Human Relations Council. Subsequent to her job with D.O. she was employed by the Medical Care and Research Foundation and worked with seniors to promote the maintenance of independent living. Her interests included music (composing), photography, travel and bridge. She had four near-grown children.

In 1981 Stevie lived on an island in Greece for one year to assist in the renovation of a friend's 150-year-old mansion. For the next eighteen summers they ran a "Bed & Breakfast" there. Stevie spent winters in the U.S.A. and worked with post-trauma clients. Since 2001 she has lived in Colorado, continually challenged by her border collie's need for go, fetch, take "jobs." She is a self-employed professional caregiver. She has five grandchildren.

Dorothy Williams Lowrie ("D.O.") is a graduate of Staten Island Academy and of Wellesley College, 1948, with a major in psychology. After marrying, she taught in elementary schools in Baltimore for two years, and moved to the Denver area in 1956. At the time of her stroke she was active as a volunteer with United Way and as a state-wide lobbyist for the Colorado League of Women Voters. She continued as a United Way volunteer after her stroke, and volunteered at the Medical Care and Research Foundation. Her interests included ceramics, duplicate bridge, cultural activities, and travel. Her husband was a Vice President of the Martin Marietta Co. in charge of the Viking Program. They had three grown children.

In 1982 the Lowries moved to Florida. Her husband was President of a division of Martin Marietta for four years. D.O. assumed the roles attendant to his new position and served on the boards of the Art Museum and the PBS T.V. and radio stations. They now live in a retirement community enjoying bridge and backgammon. D.O. has a trainer twice weekly to minimize right limb atrophy. They have three grandchildren.

133